How to Request a Test

How to Request a Test

A Clinician's Guide to the Interpretation and Evaluation of Medical Tests

Tom Boyles

Honorary Associate Professor, London School of Hygiene and Tropical Medicine, London, United Kingdom

Researcher, Clinical HIV Research Unit, University of the Witwatersrand, Johannesburg, South Africa

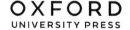

OXFORD
UNIVERSITY PRESS

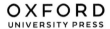

OXFORD
UNIVERSITY PRESS

Great Clarendon Street, Oxford, OX2 6DP,
United Kingdom

Oxford University Press is a department of the University of Oxford.
It furthers the University's objective of excellence in research, scholarship,
and education by publishing worldwide. Oxford is a registered trade mark of
Oxford University Press in the UK and in certain other countries

© Oxford University Press 2023

The moral rights of the author have been asserted

First Edition published in 2023

Impression: 1

Published in the United States of America by Oxford University Press
198 Madison Avenue, New York, NY 10016, United States of America

British Library Cataloguing in Publication Data

Data available

Library of Congress Control Number: 2022943242

ISBN 978-0-19-286661-5

DOI: 10.1093/med/9780192866615.001.0001

Printed and bound by
CPI Group (UK) Ltd, Croydon, CR0 4YY

Oxford University Press makes no representation, express or implied, that the
drug dosages in this book are correct. Readers must therefore always check
the product information and clinical procedures with the most up-to-date
published product information and data sheets provided by the manufacturers
and the most recent codes of conduct and safety regulations. The authors and
the publishers do not accept responsibility or legal liability for any errors in the
text or for the misuse or misapplication of material in this work. Except where
otherwise stated, drug dosages and recommendations are for the non-pregnant
adult who is not breast-feeding

Links to third party websites are provided by Oxford in good faith and
for information only. Oxford disclaims any responsibility for the materials
contained in any third party website referenced in this work.

For Robert Graham Boyles, 1935–2022.

Preface

I didn't write this book because I am an expert on the topic, I wrote it because after more than two decades of thinking and reading about the subject, I finally feel that I can convey my knowledge in the way I would like to have learned it from the beginning. In short, it is a book I wish was in my coat pocket as a medical student and junior doctor.

Testing is ubiquitous in medicine and the task of requesting tests often falls to the most junior members of the team, despite being vitally important and extremely costly. In many settings, requesting tests is a simple matter of filling out a form, ticking any number of boxes, and leaving the rest to phlebotomists, radiographers, and laboratory staff. While this has freed up junior doctors' time, it can lead to a laissez-faire attitude to testing.

As an intern, it was important to have a range of test results written in the notes as a post-intake ward round approached. Woe betide anyone who did not have a troponin result for a patient with chest pain or an amylase for a patient with abdominal pain. However, I quickly realized that experienced clinicians barely looked at some of my tests, particularly on follow-up rounds when I thought a new and pristine set of results was a core part of my job. They saw no value in my multiple C-reactive protein tests to check that a patient was recovering from pneumonia, for example, instead being happy with a brief history, examination, and inspection of the vitals chart. At the time this puzzled me and I began reading about the application of medical tests and particularly Bayes' theorem. Gradually I built up an understanding of why and when we do tests and, importantly, when not to do them.

Now I have gained a degree of experience, particularly within my specialty of infectious diseases, I see the errors I made being repeated. Typically, it is an over-reliance on tests or an overestimation of their value. Often, when doctors are unsure of the diagnosis, they request a broad range of tests in the hope that some abnormal result will lead them in the right direction. While there are some tests that are indicated for almost all patients, such as a full blood count for a patient admitted under medicine or surgery, there should be no such thing as 'routine bloods'. As a consultant, I am frequently presented with pages of blood test results that I have very little if any interest in reading. To make matters worse, sometimes the single key test I really want is not there. Sometimes I am asked to review a patient simply because a test result is 'abnormal' rather than because there is a specified clinical problem: 'We measured the beta-D-glucan [a component of the cell wall of some fungi] and it's high, please tell us which fungus the patient has' is a typical question to infectious diseases. The oncologist might similarly be faced with 'We requested a panel of tumour markers and one is elevated, come and treat this patient's cancer'. These are typical examples of performing tests without thinking through the problem in advance, and without having a full understanding of the strengths and weaknesses of the tests at hand.

The appropriate steps in evaluating and applying a new medicine is usually taught well in medical schools and most medical students and junior doctors could tell you about the four phases of clinical trials and that regulatory approval typically occurs after phase III trials confirm efficacy and safety. The same cannot be said for the evaluation of tests; this is partly because even experts disagree on the framework for test evaluation, but also because it is perceived as having less value. After reading this book, my hope is that medical students and junior doctors will have a greater appreciation of how to use tests efficiently and effectively. The quantity of tests they request is likely to decrease, which will save time and money, while the quality will increase, improving patient care.

Acknowledgements

This book would not have been possible without the love and support of my family. I would like to thank my partner, Lynne, and our two wonderful children, Maya and Kai, for putting up with me while I wrote it.

The staff at Oxford University Press have been helpful and supportive throughout, particular thanks go to Nicola Wilson for all the effort she has put in.

A number of people kindly reviewed earlier drafts and gave constructive feedback, I'd like to thank Druin Burch, Joe Wilson, Evie Rothwell, and Hywel Jones. The latter introduced me to Bayes' theorem on a ward round circa 1998, when I was a medical student—thank you for setting me on this path.

Contents

Abbreviations

ALT	alanine transaminase
AST	aspartate transaminase
AUC	area under the curve
AUROC	area under the receiver operator characteristic
BNP	brain natriuretic peptide
CA	cancer antigen
CAP	community-acquired pneumonia
COPD	chronic obstructive pulmonary disease
CrAg	cryptococcal antigen
CSF	cerebrospinal fluid
CT	computed tomography
CXR	chest X-ray
FDA	Food and Drug Administration
FHS	Framingham Heart Study
FRS	Framingham Risk Score
GP	general practitioner
HCG	human chorionic gonadotropin
HIA	Head Injury Assessment
IUGR	intrauterine growth retardation
LAM	lipoarabinomannan
LR+ve	positive likelihood ratio
LR−ve	negative likelihood ratio
MCV	mean cell volume
ML	machine learning
MPM	multivariable prediction model
MRI	magnetic resonance imaging
PCR	polymerase chain reaction
PSA	prostate-specific antigen
PTH	parathyroid hormone
ROC	receiver operator characteristic
SARS-CoV-2	severe acute respiratory syndrome coronavirus 2
STARD	Standards for Reporting Diagnostic accuracy studies
TB	tuberculosis
TBM	tuberculous meningitis
TPP	target product profile
TSH	thyroid-stimulating hormone
WHO	World Health Organization

1
Introduction

The Shrewd Professor

The general practitioner (GP) referral letter described an 18-year-old woman with 6 months of secondary amenorrhea, a negative urinary pregnancy test, and a raised prolactin level. It ended with a single-word question: prolactinoma? The on-call medical team were excited. Could this be something out of the ordinary, a break from chronic obstructive pulmonary disease (COPD) exacerbations and strokes? A slam-dunk indication for a magnetic resonance imaging (MRI) scan of the brain and a neurosurgical opinion?

Further questioning revealed that the woman had a male sexual partner and had been having regular intercourse. She stopped her oral contraception 3 months ago because she was concerned about the amenorrhea and hadn't been using alternative contraception; she had no obvious loss of libido or changes in her vision. Clinical examination including visual field testing was normal. The medical registrar requested tests for every pituitary hormone he could think of and filled out the forms for an MRI scan of the brain.

On the post-intake ward round, the professor reviewed the case. After speaking to the woman, she asked for a repeat urinary pregnancy test. The result was positive. The junior medical team were surprised and now unsure of whether the patient was pregnant or had prolactinoma; 'What should we do now?' they asked. Perhaps a serum beta-human chorionic gonadotropin (HCG) test would resolve the issue, or an ultrasound of the uterus to see if there was a visible fetus.

'Nothing', replied the professor before calmly informing the woman that she was pregnant, asking the team to cancel all the blood tests and the MRI, and moving to the next patient.

This is a true story and the medical registrar was me. I was perplexed by what had just happened; surely the GP was on to something when she found a raised prolactin in a non-pregnant woman with secondary amenorrhea? Surely the diagnosis was still in doubt, after all, there was still that negative pregnancy test? After 20 years of thinking about problems like this, I now have some understanding of what was in the professor's mind. How she was so sure about the diagnosis when the rest of us were scratching our heads.

The aim of this book is to unpack scenarios like this one: to explain how to think through the process of making such a diagnosis and, crucially, to learn what was going on in the professor's head. Whether she knew it or not, she was following a thought process based on the work of an 18th-century clergyman called Thomas Bayes. We will return to this scenario at the end of the book, when you will be able to clearly see how the professor came to a rapid and accurate diagnosis with minimal fuss and expense.

What Is a Medical Test?

For the purposes of this book, I will use a very broad definition of a medical test:

> Any procedure(s) that **elicits new information** about a patient with the intention of **improving their medical care**.

This is broad, as we can get new information in many ways: by taking a history, physical examination, direct tests (e.g. blood pressure), *in vitro* tests of patient samples, imaging, and a range of other 'special' investigations, any of which might be considered tests. We can also improve medical care in a multitude of ways—it might be something we say to a patient in terms of prognosis or advice, which medications we prescribe and at what dose, or which further tests are required. It might even be reducing delays in time to diagnosis to decrease anxiety and improve outcomes.

If you accept this broad definition, then medical testing begins the moment you first set eyes on a patient. While any number of abnormalities are possible, even when none are apparent you get a sense, but not a completely accurate picture, of the patient's age, sex/gender, height, weight, and race, which might inform you about their current or future state of health.

The next test is often a greeting in a patient's native language. For an English speaker, you might start with 'Hello!' The response of 'Hello!' would suggest functioning hearing, speech recognition, speech production, and social engagement. An absent or alternative response might represent dysfunction in any of those areas.

Only later do you start with procedures that are more traditionally considered tests, such as blood pressure measurement, physical examination, and sending samples to a laboratory, but seen in this way, any patient encounter can be viewed as a series of tests beginning with observations and ending when no more information is required.

When Are Tests Required?

The standard model for diagnosis taught in medical schools throughout the world is to begin with taking a history, then perform a physical examination, and define a differential diagnosis. Tests are then requested to refine the differential diagnosis until only one is left.

In fact, seminal research in the 1970s showed that this approach is not what practitioners do in reality.[1,2] A 1979 study of 630 medical outpatients found that the diagnosis was secure after taking a history in 56% of patients, performing an examination increased this to 73%, 'routine' investigations to 78%, and 'special' investigations to 96%.[3] A study in 2000 had similar findings with history securing the diagnosis in 79% of patients, physical examination increasing this to 87%, and investigations to 100%.[4] These studies are old and only relate to diagnosis, they say nothing about prognostic or monitoring tests, but they are likely still valid. A study from 2009[5] showed that GPs begin considering the diagnosis immediately on encountering the patient and in around 25% of cases make a 'spot diagnosis' based on something as simple as an obvious rash or barking cough. Further history taking and examination yields a diagnosis in around 50% of patients. For the rest, either no diagnostic label can be applied (10%) or further testing is required in the form of a laboratory test, a trial of treatment, or the test of time.

It is clear that clinicians can gather much of the information they require with a thoughtful history and skilful examination and laboratory tests are merely the jam in the doughnut. Junior doctors should not feel obliged to request tests just because that's what they see other doctors doing and there should be no such thing as 'routine bloods' or a 'septic screen'. Instead, there should be a careful consideration of the need for any test before the request is made. Junior doctors need to establish their own norms, and good ones, because the point of being a junior is to learn how to become senior.

Whom Do We Test?

We perform tests on populations and on individuals. Tests on populations for things like epidemiological studies, disease surveillance, and research won't be covered in this book, although many excellent resources are available. Instead, we will focus on tests we perform on individuals for their own benefit, which you are likely to use while working as a clinician. We occasionally perform tests on individuals for other people's benefit—think of an autopsy—and similar rules apply. Some argue that screening tests can only be applied to populations rather than individuals. While there is some merit to this view, we do perform, and more importantly interpret, screening tests on individuals and this will be discussed in later chapters.

Why Do We Do Tests?

This deliberately naïve question was asked to my group at medical school. The first person to answer said 'To make a diagnosis'; no doubt the lecturer was expecting this and gave a lukewarm response. He argued that we rarely do tests to make a diagnosis and preferred answers such as 'To monitor treatment response' or 'To provide a prognosis'.

Tests of individuals are often categorized with terms like diagnostic, prognostic, monitoring, early detection, risk classification, treatment selection, surveillance after treatment, and screening, but this isn't always helpful as many fit into multiple categories. Think of a biopsy as a diagnostic test for cancer—while it may confirm the diagnosis, it will also likely provide some prognostic information such as the grade of the tumour. Some tests even include a therapeutic component—think of an upper gastrointestinal endoscopy for haematemesis, which can not only diagnose the problem but provide treatment (e.g. banding of varices or injection of a bleeding ulcer).

The unifying reason we do tests on individuals, in my view, is **to answer patient-relevant questions**. The importance of this point cannot be overstated and will be a recurrent theme of this book. Every single time you request[*] a test, you should be able to formulate a patient-relevant question (or questions) in your mind remembering that **tests elicit new information about a patient with the intention of improving their medical care.**

Patient-relevant questions have two parts: the 'What?' and the 'Why?' What do you want to know and why do you want to know it? 'Does this woman with fatigue have low haemoglobin?' is only the first part as it doesn't ask why you want to know the answer. The complete question is 'Does this woman with fatigue have low haemoglobin because if so, I can search for reversible causes to treat, such as iron deficiency, and if not, I can perform other tests to search for the cause, such as thyroid function' This will be obvious to you in such a simple example and can often go unsaid, although you should be prepared to give the extended version in an exam. As a junior doctor you are likely at some point to be sent to the radiology department to request an expensive and time-consuming test like an MRI scan. If you don't want to be sent away with a flea in your ear, it is vital to know both the 'What?' and the 'Why?' of the patient-relevant question. If you aren't sure, ask your seniors for guidance. In short, when requesting a test, keep the age-old question in mind: 'Might[†] it change your management?'

Tests are often complex and answer multiple questions at the same time. You will probably request a full blood count for the woman with fatigue. While your primary question relates to the haemoglobin, you are essentially saving time for limited financial cost by asking follow-up questions in advance. If the haemoglobin is low, the first value you will look at is the mean cell volume (MCV) as it holds important information about the cause of the low haemoglobin. Further follow-up questions might be about the white cell and platelet counts, which you also get from your full blood count.

While a full blood count might answer a dozen or so questions, a complex imaging study might answer hundreds. Take the example of a 55-year-old male with cardiovascular disease and abdominal pain radiating to the back. You request a computed tomography (CT) scan of the abdomen with contrast, with the primary question,

---

[*] You request tests, you do not order them.

[†] Not all tests have to change patient management, it is acceptable to request a test where only certain results will change management.

'Does this man have a leaking abdominal aortic aneurysm, because he may require a life-saving surgical intervention?' There are associated and highly relevant follow-up questions such as whether the renal arteries are involved and perhaps anatomical details useful in planning surgery. However, the CT scan does not only look at the arteries, it also images the other abdominal organs and lung bases and it is not uncommon to find answers to questions you weren't initially considering. For example, you might find a spiculated mass at the lung base with metastases in the liver—while tragic for the patient, this unexpected finding may alter the decision regarding surgery.

Some tests answer questions that are only relevant in the future. For example, culture for tuberculosis (TB) can take up to 6 weeks to become positive. This is generally too slow to be useful in deciding whether or not to offer treatment but is sometimes vital information **after** 6 weeks of treatment. If a patient develops a drug-induced liver injury, the first question to ask is 'Does she really have TB, because if not I can stop all the treatment permanently, and if she does then I need to treat her TB in the face of the liver injury?' At this point, the culture becomes relevant: if positive, TB is confirmed, and if negative, it is in doubt. So, while requesting a culture at the time of diagnosis does not immediately answer a patient-relevant question, there is a real possibility of it becoming useful in 6 weeks' time and it might therefore be justified.

Why Learn About Tests?

The reason we need to be skilled at requesting tests is because of the costs, which must be weighed against proposed benefits when a testing decision is made. Cost can be divided into financial, direct clinical, and indirect clinical costs.

The financial cost of tests is vast. In 2006, in England alone the budget for pathology services was around £2 billion. This consisted of >500 million biochemistry and >130 million haematology tests, >50 million microbiology requests, >13 million histopathology slides, and 1 million cytology slides. A review identified that 25% of these tests were unnecessary, resulting in considerable wastage.[6] Several studies indicate that unnecessary tests account for between 25% and 40% of laboratory workload[7] and in one study, 68% of tests performed in a medical department were not considered to have contributed towards management of patients.[8] The picture is similar in the US where laboratory medicine is the single highest volume medical activity in healthcare and demand for laboratory testing is increasing disproportionately to medical activity. From 1985 to 2015, the number of laboratory tests available to clinicians more than doubled, to at least 3500.[9] The global *in vitro* diagnostics market, valued at $49 billion in 2012, represents 3–5% of all healthcare costs.

One marker of inappropriate testing comes from the variability between regions. The publication in England of the National Health Service 'Atlas of Variation' series[10] demonstrated the variation in ordering rates for diagnostic tests across 151 primary care organizations. There may be valid reasons to explain some of the observed variation, such as different populations or case mix, incidence of deprivation, disease prevalence, local policy decisions on specific services, and the availability of relatively new or high-technology tests. However, despite these factors, the variation in ordering rates is so large that it must reflect considerable differences in the individual ordering patterns of doctors within each primary care organization. For example, there was an 89-fold difference in ordering rates for brain natriuretic peptide (BNP) between different primary care organizations (Fig. 1.1). This may represent failure of guideline uptake or the unavailability of the test in some areas due to cost pressures, but is most

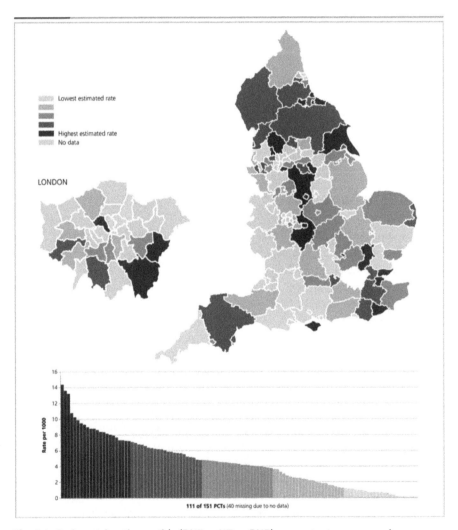

Fig. 1.1 Brain natriuretic peptide (BNP or NTproBNP) request rates across primary care organizations (primary care trusts (PCTs)) in England in 2012. From National Health Service 'Atlas of Variation'.

likely driven by both under- and over-requesting of tests by GPs. This is likely to have had significant effects on patient morbidity and mortality as well as costs.

When working in a medical system with finite resources, clearly a significant amount of money could be freed up for other services if test requests were optimized.

The direct clinical costs, or harms of tests, are typically self-evident, for example, many radiological studies require ionizing radiation. More extreme risks come with more invasive procedures, such as a brain biopsy requiring general anaesthesia and opening of the skull, which clearly comes with significant clinical risks.

Indirect clinical costs, however, are not always apparent and generally occur as a result of misinterpreting results or of finding answers to questions you didn't intend to ask. The following is a summary of a case report published in the *South African Medical Journal* showing how the misinterpretation of a new test potentially led to the demise of a patient[11]:

> The World Health Organization (WHO) recommends the Xpert MTB/RIF* as the first test of cerebrospinal fluid (CSF) from patients with suspected tuberculous meningitis (TBM). A 43-year-old HIV-positive man presented with 2 weeks of headache, recent onset of slurred speech, inability to walk, and impaired consciousness. A CT brain scan showed mild hydrocephalus and basal enhancement. CSF was yellow, with lymphocytes 300/mL, protein 1.06 g/L, and glucose 1.3 mmol/L. The Xpert MTB/RIF was negative. The admitting doctor discounted the diagnosis of TBM and prescribed ceftriaxone. The patient deteriorated and died 4 days later.

The patient was being cared for by an inexperienced clinician who had recently gained access to the Xpert MTB/RIF test and knew that it was endorsed by WHO as the first test to be undertaken when TBM is suspected. They interpreted the negative result as meaning that TBM was excluded in this patient and bacterial meningitis was more likely. An experienced clinician would have known that the clinical picture was highly suggestive of TBM and that the Xpert MTB/RIF test is not accurate enough to rule it out so would have initiated therapy immediately. Had the test not been available to the inexperienced clinician, they may well have noted that the history, examination, CSF, and brain imaging were all consistent with TBM, and initiated appropriate therapy timeously. So, in this example, providing an inexperienced clinician with an imperfect test potentially caused harm to the patient.

Other indirect costs can be finding abnormalities that were not anticipated and are of uncertain significance. It is not uncommon to find an isolated mass attached to kidneys and adrenal glands, sometimes called an 'incidentaloma', which can cause uncertainty and distress to a patient even if it is of no clinical significance.

So while tests with negligible financial and direct clinical costs may seem harmless, if they are put in the hands of inexperienced clinicians, which is commonly the case,

---

* Xpert MTB/RIF is a polymerase chain reaction (PCR)-based test for *Mycobacterium tuberculosis* DNA.

they can lead to severe unintended consequences, and may provide information that is harmful to patient care.

What Is (and Isn't) in the Book?

Although tests can be questions or examination findings, in general we will discuss *in vitro* laboratory tests and radiology, beginning when the technical aspects have been finalized. For a laboratory test, technical aspects are called analytical performance and include analytical sensitivity and specificity, limit of detection and quantitation, measurement range, linearity, metrological traceability, measurement accuracy (imprecision and trueness), and consideration of pre-analytical variables including interferences and cross-reactions. For a radiology test it would include technical aspects of exposure and image generation. I will not be discussing these technical aspects, rather I will assume that these have been satisfactorily completed and the tests have been approved for in-human testing.*

We begin in Chapter 2 by discussing diagnostic accuracy studies, which ask the fundamental question 'How accurate is this test?' Chapters 3–5 discuss the output of diagnostic accuracy studies, beginning with the most well-known but least useful (sensitivity and specificity), followed by predictive values, and finally the least well-known but most useful outputs (likelihood ratios). Chapter 6 discusses thresholds for decision-making, which provide a framework for answering the question 'Should I request this test or not?'

In Chapter 7 we change tack by stepping back from individuals to ask how tests should be evaluated beyond diagnostic accuracy studies. In Chapter 8 we discuss integrated diagnostic and prognostic research including the use of machine learning and in Chapter 9 how these diagnostic strategies can be tested in controlled trials. Chapter 10 provides some contemporary examples of how tests have been evaluated and we conclude by returning to the shrewd professor, to see how she arrived at her swift and accurate diagnosis.

Throughout the book I draw upon examples that you are likely to come across in your work as a clinician. I also tend to make up extreme examples as a way of illustrating specific points.

How to Read This Book

I understand that readers will have different levels of background knowledge, of interest in the subject, and of time to spend on the book. Each chapter therefore

---

* The story of Theranos from the book Bad Blood: Secrets and Lies in a Silicon Valley Startup by John Carreyrou is an accessible way to read about the trials and tribulations of attempting to develop new tests for regulatory approval.

begins with core knowledge, generally describing simpler scenarios with multiple convenient assumptions that may not be applicable in all real-world settings. Some chapters also have advanced knowledge sections to take the reader a little further into the subject and typically tackle scenarios where assumptions used in basic models no longer apply. My hope is that by reading all the core sections, a reader will get a basic understanding of the concepts contained in the book, with the understanding that real-life scenarios may be more complex. The advanced knowledge sections will be an introduction to more realistic scenarios for the curious.

⊙ See Video 1—Introduction—available at:
https://doi.org/10.1093/med/9780192866615.012.0001.

Notes

1. Elstein AS, Kagan N, Shulman LS, Jason H, Loupe MJ. Methods and theory in the study of medical inquiry. J Med Educ. 1972;47(2):85–92.
2. Elstein AS, Shulman LS, Sprafka SA. Medical problem-solving. J Med Educ. 1981;56(1):75–76.
3. Sandler G. Costs of unnecessary tests. Br Med J. 1979;2(6181):21–24.
4. Roshan M, Rao AP. A study on relative contributions of the history, physical examination and investigations in making medical diagnosis. J Assoc Physicians India. 2000;48(8):771–775.
5. Heneghan C, Glasziou P, Thompson M, Rose P, Balla J, Lasserson D, et al. Diagnostic strategies used in primary care. BMJ. 2009;338:b946.
6. Lord Carter of Coles. Report of the Second Phase of the Review of NHS Pathology Services in England. An Independent Review for the Department of Health. Report No. 291710. London: Department of Health; 2008.
7. Rao GG, Crook M, Tillyer ML. Pathology tests: is the time for demand management ripe at last? J Clin Pathol. 2003;56(4):243–248.
8. Miyakis S, Karamanof G, Liontos M. Factors contributing to inappropriate ordering of tests in an academic medical department and the effect of an educational feedback strategy. Postgrad Med J. 2006;82(974):823–829.
9. Freedman DB. Towards better test utilization—strategies to improve physician ordering and their impact on patient outcomes. EJIFCC. 2015;26(1):15–30.
10. Office for Health Improvement and Disparities. Atlas of variation. Available at: https://fingertips.phe.org.uk/profile/atlas-of-variation
11. Bhigjee A. Use of the Xpert MTB/RIF assay in the diagnosis of tuberculous meningitis: a cautionary note. S Afr Med J. 2014;104(10):650.

2
Determining the Accuracy of a Test

Once a test has achieved acceptable analytical performance in the laboratory and has been approved for use in clinical practice, a reasonable first question is 'How accurate is it?' The answer comes from accuracy studies, which may be diagnostic or prognostic. Accuracy studies are relatively cheap to perform and help researchers or developers decide which tests should go forward to the next phase of evaluation.

A diagnostic accuracy study evaluates the ability of one or more medical tests (known as the **index test(s)**) to correctly classify study participants as having a **target condition** or not. This is done by comparing the distribution of the index test results with those of a **reference standard** in a well-defined **population and setting**.

As with all evidence-based medicine, to perform a high-quality accuracy study we begin with a question, which includes each of these terms. For example, if we wish to know the diagnostic accuracy of a new urinary pregnancy test, the question might be 'In women buying urinary pregnancy (**target condition**) tests for themselves at a commercial pharmacy (**population and setting**), what is the diagnostic accuracy of "a novel test" (**index test**) compared to ultrasound of the uterus (**reference test**)?' We will consider each of these terms in turn before considering the output of accuracy studies.

Target Condition

The target condition, which might be a disease, a disease stage, a response or benefit from therapy, or an event or condition in the future, must be clearly defined in advance. In many instances this might be unambiguous, for example, pregnancy. At other times it must be clearly defined, for example, stage 4 malignancy might need to be defined as disease that has spread from its origin to distant parts of the body. The target condition doesn't necessarily have to be present right now, it could be in the future, for example, a prognostic test to determine the future risk of stroke.

Index Tests

An index test is any method for collecting information about the current or future health status of a patient and can be an imaging procedure, a laboratory test, elements from history and physical examination, or a combination of these. The simplest

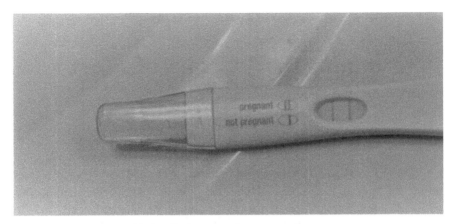

Fig. 2.1 Urinary lateral flow assay for pregnancy.

example would be a laboratory test with a binary (positive or negative) outcome such as a lateral flow assay with a control line and a test line (Fig. 2.1). So long as the control line is present, the result is positive when the test line appears and negative when it does not.

Many tests don't give binary outcomes; rather, the results are either continuous (numbers or ratios) or ordinal (more than two categories). When values are continuous, it may be appropriate to choose a threshold value above which it is considered positive and below, negative. For example, when measuring serum beta-HCG to determine pregnancy, there is a threshold value above which it is considered positive and below, negative; this should always be determined in advance.

Some lateral flow assays even give ambiguous results. Lipoarabinomannan (LAM) is a highly conserved protein in the cell wall of *Mycobacterium tuberculosis*, the causative organism of TB. LAM can be detected in urine using a lateral flow device but rather than giving a definitive '+ve' or '−ve' signal, the degree of colour change of the test line is dependent on the concentration of LAM in the urine. The manufacturers supply a test card to compare with the actual test and it requires a degree of judgement by the observer to determine the test result.

It is therefore important to consider who is interpreting the index test. Ideally, it will be the person interpreting it in the real-world scenario. For a home pregnancy test, it would be the women in the study who have read the instructions. For a laboratory test, it would use the same standard operating procedures that will be used when the test is rolled out. For tests like LAM, it is usual for two experienced laboratory technicians to independently read each test and when results are discrepant, a third reader is used. This is fine if the same approach will be used when the test is rolled out; however, in this particular example, LAM may be used by clinicians at the bedside rather than technicians in a laboratory so it would be important either to use clinician interpretation for the accuracy study or at least validate clinician interpretation against technician interpretation in a separate study.

Many tests are far harder to interpret than a lateral flow assay. We sometimes say that the results are operator dependent. Think of an ultrasound scan when the operator is manipulating the probe to obtain the image and simultaneously interpreting the results; this is clearly a skill which varies between operators and it is vital that the experience level of the operators is clearly recorded. It is also important that clear criteria and definitions of pathology are determined in advance.

In summary, interpretation of the index test should be as close to real-world conditions as possible with all outcomes determined a priori and fully disclosed in the report.

Reference Standards

A reference standard is the best available method for establishing the presence or absence of the target condition and the choice is critical to the validity of an accuracy study. The reference standard is sometimes called the 'gold standard' or 'ground truth'; I avoid the term 'gold standard' as it implies that the reference standard is perfect and will never change. In reality, reference standards are arrived at by consensus and are therefore subject to differences of opinion and can change over time as new and improved technologies become available. Sometimes, consensus opinion might be that no 100% accurate reference standard exists, or imperfect reference standards may be necessary due to cost, practical considerations, or because of risk to participants.

Consider the example of the reference standard for first-trimester pregnancy which is needed to study a novel urinary pregnancy test (the index test). One might consider a number of possibilities; the simplest and cheapest might be an established urinary pregnancy test even if it is known not to give the correct result every time. A better, but more expensive choice might be serum beta-HCG as it is known that measuring the 'pregnancy hormone' in the blood rather than the urine is more likely to give the correct answer. Better still might be an ultrasound of the uterus, as the finding of a fetus with a beating heart confirms pregnancy, although it remains operator dependent and may be negative in very early pregnancy. Even better than one ultrasound might be two ultrasounds 3 months apart, repeating the test helps to exclude operator dependency and excludes the uncertainty in very early pregnancy. Even so, it could be argued that even performing two ultrasound scans 3 months apart is not a perfect reference standard. Consider an extra-uterine pregnancy, finding a fetus without a heartbeat, a molar pregnancy, or a woman who actually became pregnant or aborted a fetus between the scans. Any of these might challenge our assumptions that the reference standard is perfect.

In this example, there are a number of choices of reference standard which are likely to get closer and closer to the perfect reference standard we are looking for but also to be increasingly costly. In practice, we should use the agreed best reference standard we can afford, report exactly what was used, and acknowledge any limitations.

In some instances, the reference standard is far more difficult to choose and apply. Take the example of TBM. While not always possible or practical, the ideal reference standard for an infectious disease is to grow (culture) the causative organism from a sterile patient specimen. In this case culturing *M. tuberculosis* (causative organism) from CSF (sterile patient specimen) confirms the diagnosis. The problem is that we know from autopsy studies that patients who definitely have TBM can have negative CSF cultures. Autopsy is clearly not a practical reference standard and so we are left with the problem of which reference standard to use when CSF culture is negative. The solution in this case is that a group of top TBM researchers had a meeting where they sat and discussed definitions of TBM for research purposes and then published them in an academic journal. The researchers agreed that the definitions were not perfect but that by applying the same definitions in different research studies, it would be easy to compare their work with each other.

A particular type of reference standard that you will see every day when working as a junior doctor are reference ranges that are provided with most continuous results from laboratory tests. Reference ranges can have lower or upper boundaries but most commonly have both. For example, the typical reference range for plasma sodium is 135–145 mmol/L. It is important to understand how the values are calculated and how to use them to interpret your test results. Laboratory scientists go to great lengths to provide us with useful reference values and it is not easy. A basic method might be to select a large group of 'healthy people', measure the analyte in question, and plot the results; assuming a normal distribution, the reference range might be quoted as two standard deviations either side of the mean. The difficulties and limitations of such a method are fairly clear—you would need to define 'healthy people' and would need to use exactly the same specimen collection and laboratory methods as the real-world setting. The reference range would then only apply to people within the domain of 'healthy people' you chose, a group with different biological sex, ethnicity, age, and so on might produce different values. Even then you would be left with a reference range where 5% of 'healthy people' had an 'abnormal' value; based on this alone, you might expect 1 in 20 of all tests on a perfectly healthy person to fall outside the reference range. Clearly, reference ranges are challenging to develop and must be used with caution by the clinician.

Population and Setting

The choice of population and setting for an accuracy study is also critical to its validity. The very first studies of a novel diagnostic might use a case-controlled design—these have the advantage of being cheap and convenient but are very weak evidence that a test will be useful in a real-world setting. A case-controlled design involves selecting a group of patients or samples who definitely have the condition (reference standard positive) and a group who definitely do not have the condition (reference standard negative), then applying the index test to these groups. Often these types of studies are performed on samples that have been stored in laboratories for convenience and cost reduction.

Imagine this extreme example. You have developed a new super quick and cheap urinary pregnancy test and want to see how well it works, so you go to an antenatal clinic where 10-week dating scans are being performed. You select female/male couples leaving the room with smiling faces as you are pretty sure that one will be pregnant and the other not. You perform the new test on 50 couples and determine that your test has excellent accuracy in differentiating pregnant from non-pregnant people. Should you be ecstatic and begin marketing your test?

It's pretty obvious that the answer is no.

In fact, any test that can reliably differentiate females from males will perform pretty well in these circumstances. A reliable measure of testosterone levels would work pretty well. A level above 150 ng/dL would indicate not being pregnant (normal range for men 240–950 ng/dL) and a level below 150 ng/dL would indicate pregnancy (normal range for women 8–60 ng/dL). While the test might make the odd error, with, for example, a transgender man, it would otherwise be pretty accurate at determining pregnancy in an antenatal clinic but it should be obvious that it would be terrible in a population of women who want to know whether or not they are pregnant.

While a case-controlled study might be worth performing because a test that performs badly can be discarded without wasting significant resources, a test that performs well has only jumped the lowest of hurdles on the way to being used in the real world. Of course, not all case-controlled studies are as extreme as my example, but it is important to be aware that when you read a diagnostic accuracy study, positive case-controlled studies are very weak evidence that a test will be useful in the real world.

A preferred but more expensive trial design is an observational cohort accuracy study. Rather than selecting patients or samples based on the presence or absence of a condition, the study begins by selecting an unbiased sample of patients for whom the test is intended to be used in future—this is known as the **domain**. In the case of the novel urinary pregnancy test, this might be women buying tests for themselves at a representative sample of pharmacies. To reduce the potential level of bias in the sample, it is important to either sample participants at random or in consecutive order that they present. Any form of non-random sampling (e.g. only people who respond to an advert are included in the study), while necessary in some cases, introduces unwanted bias.

In the case of a new test for TBM, it might be a consecutive or random sample of patients admitted to hospital with chronic headache and clinical features of meningitis. From a medical perspective, this would be any patient in whom TBM formed part of the differential diagnosis based on clinical criteria. Any deviation from these conditions, such as non-random sampling or inappropriate exclusions, introduces bias to the study.

Action

It is important to consider the implications of incorrect results, which can be divided into false positive (index test positive when reference standard is negative) and false negative (index test is negative when reference standard is positive), these are sometimes known as actions. False-positive results could be devastating for patients if, for example, they are diagnosed with a tumour that requires amputation of a leg, when in fact the reference standard confirms that no tumour is present. Less troubling would be falsely diagnosing a self-limiting viral upper respiratory tract infection. Similarly, false-negative index test results would be calamitous if a patient was wrongly cleared of a cancer that subsequently progressed. A false negative would have less severe consequences if the index condition was self-limiting.

Box 2.1 is an example of how these items are put together by a group of experts and is taken from a review of rapid, point-of-care antigen and molecular-based tests for diagnosis of severe acute respiratory syndrome coronavirus 2 (SARS-CoV-2) infection by the Cochrane COVID-19 Diagnostic Test Accuracy Group.[1] This group of experts clearly define the question, population, index test, target condition, reference standard, and action before proceeding to their results.

Statistical Output

The output of an accuracy study when both index and reference standards are binary is a 2×2 table (Table 2.1). Each participant can fall into any of the four boxes. By convention the letters A–D are used. We will discuss the 2×2 table extensively in Chapters 3–5 and it is worth familiarizing yourself with it now. We will discuss the interpretation of the 2×2 table in Chapter 3.

Index Tests With Continuous Outputs

In this section, we will expand on issues of index test outcomes being non-binary. As you will know, many test results are continuous (numerical) values; almost all biochemical and haematology tests are continuous, and are typically reported as the ratio of the entity we are measuring to the volume of serum or plasma (e.g. sodium is typically reported as millimoles per litre of plasma).

Imagine that endocrinologists have used a reference standard to divide a group of patients into those with and without hypothyroidism. The diagnostic (index) test is thyroid-stimulating hormone (TSH), which is a continuous variable. It is higher when patients are hypothyroid and lower when euthyroid. If TSH, or any other continuous test, was perfect, we could choose a cut-off value above which we would diagnose hypothyroidism and below which we would discount it. In real-life scenarios, this is

Box 2.1 Review of rapid, point-of-care antigen and molecular-based tests for diagnosis of SARS-CoV-2 infection by the Cochrane COVID-19 Diagnostic Test Accuracy Group

Question
What is the diagnostic accuracy of rapid point-of-care antigen and molecular-based tests for the diagnosis of SARS-CoV-2 infection?

Population
Adults or children with suspected:

- Current SARS-CoV-2 infection.

Or populations undergoing screening for SARS-CoV-2 infection, including:

- Asymptomatic contacts of confirmed COVID-19 cases.
- Community screening.

Index test
Any rapid antigen or molecular-based test for diagnosis of SARS-CoV-2 meeting the following criteria:

- Portable or mains-powered device.
- Minimal sample preparation requirements.
- Minimal biosafety requirements.
- No requirement for a temperature-controlled environment.
- Test results available within 2 hours of sample collection.

Target condition
Detection of current SARS-CoV-2 infection.

Reference standard
For COVID-19 cases: positive reverse transcription polymerase chain reaction (RT-PCR) alone or clinical diagnosis of COVID-19 based on established guidelines or combinations of clinical features.
    For non-COVID-19 cases: negative RT-PCR or pre-pandemic sources of samples.

Action
False-negative results mean missed cases of COVID-19 infection, with either delayed or no confirmed diagnosis and increased risk of community transmission due to false sense of security.
False-positive results lead to unnecessary self-isolation or quarantine, with the potential for new infection to be acquired.

Table 2.1 A 2×2 table representing the output of a diagnostic accuracy study when both reference standard and index test are binary

	Definitely has the condition	Definitely does not have the condition
Test is positive	A True positive	B False positive
Test is negative	C False negative	D True negative

very rarely the case; instead, the distribution of values for reference test positive and negative cases overlap. The degree to which they diverge is a measure of diagnostic accuracy.

Fig. 2.2 illustrates how results of a diagnostic accuracy study might look for a continuous variable such as TSH using three different assays. Each graph shows frequency distributions for those with positive and negative reference tests. The overlap between frequency distributions (shaded area) is greatest in A and decreases as we move to B and C. This suggests that A has the lowest diagnostic accuracy and C the highest.

It is important to realize that an implicit assumption in Fig. 2.2 is that the frequency distribution of index tests always approximates to a normal distribution. This may not be true in all real-life examples although the concept of overlapping frequency distributions remains sound.

Summary

- Diagnostic accuracy studies compare **index tests** of **target conditions** to **reference standards** in a defined **population and setting**.
- Index tests and target conditions must be clearly defined in advance.
- The reference standard, which might not be 100% accurate, must be chosen carefully and fully described.
- Case-controlled trial designs are cheaper and easier to perform but have limited validity.
- Diagnostic accuracy studies with high validity are performed in the same **population** and **setting (domain)** that the test will be used in practice, using random or consecutive sampling.
- The output of a diagnostic accuracy study when the index test result is binary is a 2×2 table.
- The output of a diagnostic accuracy study when the index test result is continuous can be viewed as two frequency distributions.

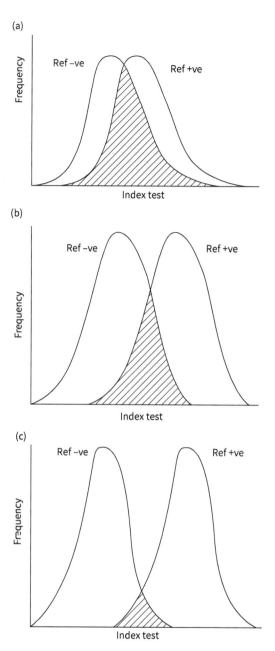

Fig. 2.2 Frequency distributions for thyroid-stimulating hormone (TSH) in patients with (right) and without (left) hypothyroidism according to a reference standard. Each graph represents a different theoretical assay with accuracy increasing from (a) to (c).

Advanced Knowledge

Consensus Guidelines

There are two important consensus guidelines which can be applied to diagnostic accuracy studies. The first is the STARD guideline, which stands for 'Standards for Reporting Diagnostic accuracy studies'. It is a list of items that researchers should include when reporting a diagnostic accuracy study. Editors and reviewers are encouraged to check that all items have been included before publishing a study. The 30 items under the headings of title or abstract, abstract, introduction, methods, results, discussion, and other information can be found at: https://www.equator-network.org/reporting-guidelines/stard/

A related tool is QUADAS-2: 'Quality Assessment of Diagnostic Accuracy Studies'. This is the recommended tool for use in systematic reviews to evaluate the risk of bias and applicability of diagnostic accuracy studies. It consists of four key domains: patient selection, index test, reference standard, and flow and timing. It can be found at: http://www.bristol.ac.uk/population-health-sciences/projects/quadas/

By examining each of these checklists you will see what is required to produce a high-quality, high-applicability study at low risk of bias.

⏺ See Video 2—Diagnostic_accuracy_studies—available at: https://doi.org/10.1093/med/9780192866615.012.0002.

Note

1. Dinnes J, Deeks JJ, Berhane S, Taylor M, Adriano A, Davenport C, et al. Rapid, point-of-care antigen and molecular-based tests for diagnosis of SARS-CoV-2 infection. Cochrane Database Syst Rev. 2021;3:CD013705.

3
Test Accuracy, Sensitivity, and Specificity

You understand how to perform a diagnostic accuracy study to arrive at a 2×2 table (Table 3.1). You also understand that the results are only as good as the study and may not necessarily be applicable to the patient you have in front of you. However, we will now move on to interpreting the 2×2 table; personally, when I think about the interpretation of an accuracy study, I bring up a mental picture of a 2×2 table in my mind and use it as an aide-memoire.

Test accuracy answers the question 'What proportion of test results are correct?' and is the simplest value we can calculate from the 2×2 table. It is defined as the total of all correct results as a proportion of all the tests performed. True positive plus true negative divided by all tests performed.

It is calculated as $(A+D)/(A+B+C+D)$.

Sensitivity answers the question 'In patients who **definitely have the condition**, what is the chance that the **test will be positive?**'

It is calculated using only the first column of the 2×2 table as $A/(A+C)$.

Specificity answers the question 'In patients who **definitely do not have the condition**, what is the chance that the **test will be negative**'

It is calculated using only the second column of the 2×2 table as $D/(B+D)$.

Test accuracy is often reported in mainstream media as it seems intuitive that the greater the accuracy, the better the test. If the media report that a test has, for example, 95% accuracy, many people would be impressed. However, this can be misleading; take the example of a test for a rare cancer with a prevalence of 1 in 1000. A test which always reads negative, regardless of the status of the patient, will be correct 999/1000 times. It would have an accuracy of 99.9% despite the test being entirely useless. In contrast, a test that is correct 80% of the time for a condition such as pneumonia with 50% prevalence in a population might turn out to be useful. Clearly, if we want to understand which tests are useful, we need a more detailed metric.

Sensitivity and specificity are rivalled only by the p-value as the most misunderstood and over-valued statistical terms in medicine.[*] However, they are widely taught and discussed among clinicians so it's important to understand them. In particular, it is important to know their limitations.

---

[*] To learn more about what p-values mean, and crucially what they don't mean, I recommend the p-value fallacy, see Goodman SN. Toward evidence-based medical statistics. 1: The P value fallacy. Ann Intern Med. 1999;130(12):995–1004.

Table 3.1 A 2×2 table representing the output of a diagnostic accuracy study when both reference standard and index test are binary

	Definitely has the condition	Definitely does not have the condition
Test is positive	A True positive	B False positive
Test is negative	C False negative	D True negative

Before going any further, ask yourself this question:

A patient wants to know what her chance is of having breast cancer. You have a test for breast cancer that has been widely researched in the population she comes from. The sensitivity is 90% and the specificity 98%. You administer the test which is positive, what is the probability that the woman has breast cancer? Multiple choice answers are:

(a) 90%.

(b) 98%.

(c) I don't know.

Think for a moment before you check the answer.

The correct answer is (c), 'I don't know'. If you answered (a) or (b) you are not alone, I have asked this question in many lectures of experienced doctors and it is uncommon for more than a quarter to get it right.

To understand the answer, think back to the 2×2 table and what questions sensitivity and specificity answer. Sensitivity is calculated from the first column and can only tell definitively about women with breast cancer (Table 3.2).

Specificity is calculated from the second column and can only tell definitively about women without breast cancer (Table 3.3).

However, the only thing we definitely know about this woman is that her test is positive, which means that she lies somewhere in the first **row**, either A or B (Table 3.4).

Table 3.2 Sensitivity is concerned only with patients who definitely have the condition, the first column of a 2×2 table

	Definitely has the condition	Definitely does not have the condition
Test is positive	A	B
Test is negative	C	D

Table 3.3 Specificity is concerned only with patients who definitely do not have the condition, the second column of a 2×2 table

	Definitely has the condition	Definitely does not have the condition
Test is positive	A	B
Test is negative	C	D

It should be obvious by now that neither sensitivity nor specificity alone can answer the patient-relevant question 'Given that I have a positive test, what is the chance that I have cancer?'

Hopefully you can see that sensitivity and specificity answer questions that we almost never ask. It would be highly unusual for a patient to ask you 'I definitely have rheumatoid arthritis, can you tell me how likely it is that my rheumatoid factor will be raised?' If that happened, you could answer with the sensitivity of the test, but the chances are it never will.

Sensitivity and Specificity Are Highly Context Dependent

You will often hear senior colleagues say things like 'The sensitivity is about 80% and the specificity is about 90%, so it's a pretty good test'. As the rest of the book will explain, this is a highly misleading statement. With a few caveats explained below, I will argue that unless sensitivity and specificity are both 100% in all circumstances, results of a diagnostic accuracy test when reported in this way are of limited value as they are highly context dependent. At this stage I will simply explain with an example.

Imagine that I offer you a new test with sensitivity 96% and specificity 96% when evaluated in high-quality diagnostic accuracy studies. It is fast, cheap, and causes no discomfort to the patient. Sounds good so far.

Now imagine that this test is for diagnosing death. Junior doctors spend quite a lot of time diagnosing death. We are taught to perform tests such as feeling for pulses,

Table 3.4 Patients with a positive test are placed in the first row of a 2×2 table

	Definitely has the condition	Definitely does not have the condition
Test is positive	A	B
Test is negative	C	D

testing corneal reflexes, and listening for heart and breath sounds. If all are negative, we diagnose death, but it isn't an exact science. Every year there are stories of people diagnosed as dead who wake up in mortuaries. It also takes a fair amount of time, so imagine a highly accurate device you point at the patient's forehead and it gives a reading 'Dead vs alive'.* This could save countless hours for harassed junior doctors, perhaps we could shift the task of diagnosing death to nurses or nursing assistants.

What do you think about the sensitivity and specificity of the highly accurate test now?

If you used it, for 1 in 25 dead people you would tell the relatives the patient was alive, and for 1 in 25 living people you would tell the relatives the patient was dead. All of a sudden, sensitivity and specificity of 96% doesn't seem so accurate after all.

Apply the same test to diagnosing rhinovirus in a patient with a runny nose and the diagnostic accuracy would probably be fine. There's no great harm in telling someone with a runny nose that they don't have rhinovirus when they do (or vice versa), so getting it wrong occasionally doesn't matter too much.

As you can see from these examples, the importance we place on a test's sensitivity and specificity depends on the clinical implications of a false result.

So should we abandon sensitivity and specificity as useless?

I think the answer is no.

When Sensitivity and Specificity Are Useful

I can think of two instances when knowing the sensitivity and specificity of a test, when calculated from high-quality accuracy studies conducted in the population from which a patient is drawn, is useful.

The first is when either sensitivity or specificity approaches 100%, that is, either false positives (B) or false negatives (C) are vanishingly rare.

Fig. 3.1 is a blood smear with *Trypanosoma* species clearly visible and is an example of a test with 100% specificity. If this test is positive, the patient definitely has trypanosomiasis (there are actually three species of human trypanosomiasis, but for the example we will assume that the patient has only been exposed to one of them). It is inconceivable that a patient without trypanosomiasis could have this test result and so the false-positive rate (B) is zero. Table 3.5 describes the test, and while we can guess at the values for A, C, and D, we can be pretty confident that B (false positives) will be zero. By knowing that, we also know any patient in the first row will fall into box A (true positive). In those patients with a negative blood smear, we remain uncertain of their status, and thus cannot exclude trypanosomiasis.

You can make a similar argument when the sensitivity is 100% in all scenarios. Tests with 100% sensitivity or specificity are typically the best available reference

---

* This would be a great test to try on Schrödinger's cat—but I digress.

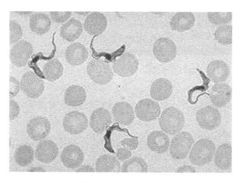

Fig. 3.1 Trypanosomes on a blood film.

standards. Tests that are both 100% sensitive and specific in all circumstances are rare and typically define the condition in question. It could be argued that measuring serum sodium is both 100% sensitive and specific for hyponatraemia as any value <135 mmol/L indicates hyponatraemia and any value ≥135 mmol/L is not hyponatraemia. This isn't surprising when the definition of hyponatraemia is serum sodium <135 mmol/L. However, even in these circumstances we need to be careful—perhaps there is an unmeasured severe hyperlipidaemia or paraproteinaemia causing pseudohyponatraemia, essentially a falsely low reading due to the presence of the lipid or protein. In real-world settings, we should also consider practical issues such as incorrect labelling of samples and faulty machines which can provide spurious results.

The aim of diagnostic tests when considering a differential diagnosis is to either rule diagnoses IN or rule them OUT. In this context, you might have heard terms such as:

- SpIN, which means tests with high Specificity are good at ruling a condition IN.
- SnOUT, which means tests with high Sensitivity are good at ruling a condition OUT.

These terms are appealing for their simplicity and memorability. They may even help you answer questions in a medical school exam, but they can also be highly

Table 3.5 The 2×2 table for blood smears in patients with and without trypanosomiasis

	Trypanosomiasis	No trypanosomiasis
Trypanosoma +ve blood smear	A	Zero
Trypanosoma −ve blood smear	C	D

misleading. Let's take a test with 85% sensitivity and 96% specificity. You would think that this was good at 'ruling in' a condition when positive. In fact, if the prevalence of the condition is 1% in the population you are sampling and the test is positive, the probability of the condition being present is only 18% (we will discuss the importance of prevalence in this calculation in Chapters 4 and 5). That's pretty terrible in most circumstances as there is a 78% chance the patient does not have the condition, even though this test with apparently good 'rule-in' value is positive.

If understanding the relevance of sensitivity and specificity when one value approaches 100% is difficult, you can imagine that when neither approaches 100% it is very difficult indeed.

There is nothing intuitive about answering the patient-relevant question 'When prevalence is 10% and a test has sensitivity of 75% and specificity of 85%, what is the probability of disease after a positive and negative test?' The answer happens to be 36% and 3% respectively, but I needed an online calculator to work it out. We will cover these calculations in Chapter 5, but at this stage it is worth remembering that while SpIN and SnOUT are easy to remember, they might not give you the answer you expect, and intuitively answering patient-relevant questions when neither sensitivity nor specificity approach 100% is close to impossible.

The second instance that sensitivity and specificity are useful is in comparing new tests with old, with the **key assumption** that the two tests are equivalent in all other ways (e.g. cost, harm to patient, and turnaround time). If, for example, an existing test has been shown to be useful with sensitivity X and specificity Y, a new test with improved sensitivity and equal specificity (or vice versa), is likely to be advantageous.* If, however, the sensitivity is higher and specificity lower (or vice versa), the new test will not automatically be an improvement.

The take-home message at this stage is that, unless at least one value is 100%, or you are comparing new tests with old, sensitivity and specificity are of limited value because they don't directly answer patient-relevant questions. Next time you hear someone confidently describe a test as 'good' because the sensitivity is, say, 80% and specificity is, say, 90%, perhaps ask them (politely) what the results mean for individual patients.

---

* Technically speaking, a test with higher specificity but the same sensitivity should always be better as it leads to withholding treatment from more patients without the condition (always a good thing), whereas a test with higher sensitivity but the same specificity leads to treatment of more people with the disease. This is likely to be a good thing if disease is homogenous (patients with the condition are similar to one another and all require the same treatment), but if the new test picks up slightly different patients than the old test, we still need to be sure that treatment is efficacious in that group. This technical point can often be ignored.

Index Tests With Continuous Outputs

Fig. 2.2 in Chapter 2 showed the frequency distributions of continuous index tests given a binary reference standard. An alternative way of presenting the same data and generating a statistic is shown in Fig. 3.2. Each curve corresponds with the frequency distribution in Fig. 2.2. Each point along the curve represents its own 2×2 table depending on the value of the index test chosen as the cut-off between positive and negative. Sensitivity on the y-axis is plotted against (1 − specificity) on the x-axis for each cut-off value. On the left, the cut-off value is highest, ensuring high specificity (very few false positives) traded off against low sensitivity (very many false negatives);

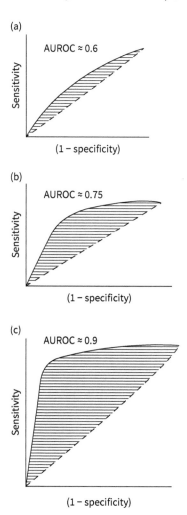

Fig. 3.2 Receiver operator characteristic (ROC) curves for TSH in patients with and without hypothyroidism according to a reference standard. Each graph represents a different theoretical assay with accuracy increasing from (a) to (c).

as you move along the curve, the cut-off value decreases and this trade-off is gradually reversed until the far right where the cut-off value is very low with correspondingly high sensitivity and low specificity. This is known as a receiver operator characteristics (ROC) curve.

The dashed line from bottom left to top right is the chance line; the ROC curve would run along that line if the frequency distributions completely overlapped and test results were no better than chance. The ROC curves in Fig. 3.2 bow out from the chance line to different degrees. Curve (a) bows out very little from the chance line, corresponding with highly overlapping frequency distributions and poor discrimination. Curve (b) bows out a little more and curve (c) more still, corresponding with decreased overlap of frequency distributions and improving discrimination.

In each of (a), (b), and (c) the area between the ROC curve and chance line is shaded. This is known as the area under the ROC curve (AUROC) or C-statistic; it is 0.5 when the ROC curve runs along the chance line (random index test results) and 1.0 for a perfect test where the ROC curve is a vertical and horizontal line. Approximate values of 0.6, 0.75, and 0.9 are given for the ROC curves in (a), (b), and (c) respectively.

ROC curves give us a unified statistic (AUROC or C-statistic) for how well a test with continuous output discriminates between patients with and without the condition and the question remains 'What is a "good" AUROC?'

There is a convention which says that 0.7–0.8 is reasonable, 0.8–0.9 is good, and >0.9 is excellent, but you will realize by now that, as with sensitivity and specificity, the interpretation of the AUROC is highly context dependent (although it may be useful to compare new tests with old).

A further limitation of ROC curves is that they tell us nothing about the prevalence of the condition. A key assumption previously was that the population is evenly split (50:50) between those with and without the condition, but this is rarely true. Typically, there are many more patients without the condition than with it, that is, most men tested for prostate cancer will not have it. This fact is not captured by an ROC curve.

AUROC values tend to be exaggerated in populations where there are far fewer people with the condition than without it. This is common, as we typically study tests in populations with a relatively low prevalence. AUROC values are typically higher in unbalanced populations compared to balanced ones, essentially because the large number of true negatives that are correctly identified inflates the value. The solution is to plot a precision–recall curve,[1] this is similar to a ROC curve but essentially ignores all the true negatives, by plotting sensitivity against positive predictive value. A test which is performed on an imbalanced population may have a high AUROC but a poor precision-recall value.

Summary

- Accuracy, sensitivity, and specificity are generated from a 2×2 table.
- These are most useful when values approach 100% or when comparing tests.

- When neither sensitivity nor specificity approach 100%, it is not intuitively obvious what test results mean for patients.
- Aside from a 100% accurate test, the concept of a 'good' sensitivity and specificity is highly context dependent.
- ROC curves summarize overlapping frequency distributions when the index test is a continuous variable.
- The AUROC (or C-statistic) summarizes diagnostic accuracy when the index test is a continuous variable.
- AUROCs give a reasonable summary of discrimination of a test when a population is balanced between those with and without the condition.
- Precision–recall curves are more informative when populations are imbalanced.

Advanced Knowledge

Why Do Sensitivity and Specificity Vary Between Studies?

Fig. 3.3 is a Forest plot taken from a systematic review.[2] Each pair of squares are the results of a diagnostic accuracy study and the lines are confidence intervals. The studies are very similar: in each case the index test is Xpert MTB/RIF, which is a PCR-based test for TB, the reference standard is culture of the same sample for *Mycobacterium tuberculosis*, the target condition is TB in the lungs (TB can occur anywhere in the body), and the population is adults with HIV infection and symptoms of TB. The main difference between studies is their settings which are in a wide variety of countries.

The first thing to strike you is that the specificity of each study is pretty high and pretty constant: the pooled specificity is 98%, with narrow 95% confidence intervals (98–99%). In contrast, the sensitivity varies enormously from a little over 40% to close to 100%, the pooled sensitivity is 77%, with wide 95% confidence intervals (71–82%). There is no pattern of sensitivity by country, they are randomly distributed. The obvious question therefore is why the range of values for sensitivity when studies are so similar, and there is no pattern based on geography?

The answer lies largely in the subtle differences between the studies. They may seem homogeneous because index test, reference standards, target condition, and population are similar but in reality, diagnostic accuracy is highly susceptible to small differences between studies, which is a major limitation. Close inspection of all 30 studies would reveal some obvious differences; for example, some studies classified patients as negative for the index test if they were unable to produce a sample of sputum, while other studies excluded such patients from evaluation. Other differences are more subtle such as differing age and biological sex profile or different proportions of patients taking antiretroviral therapy.

While the specificity of Xpert MTB/RIF seems consistent between studies, Fig. 3.4 shows that this can be misleading. It shows how the specificity of an almost identical

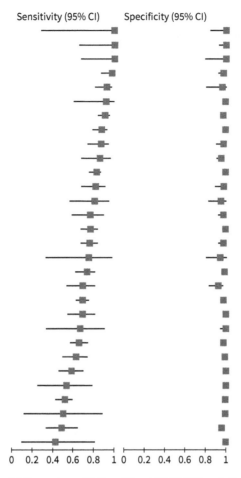

Fig. 3.3 A plot of sensitivity and specificity of Xpert MTB/RIF in adult patients with HIV suspected of having pulmonary TB. Each pair of dots represents a different study. CI, confidence interval. From Horne et al. (2019).[2]

test (Xpert MTB/RIF Ultra) varies, not between studies but between patients within the **same** study.[3] All patients have previously been treated for TB and have now returned with symptoms and are included in the accuracy study. The x-axis is time since the patient completed their previous course of antituberculous treatment and the y-axis is the specificity. The four lines represent slightly different tests and interpretations, but they convey the same message: specificity improves consistently as the time since treatment completion increases. The likely reason is that the test identifies TB DNA which can remain in patients' lungs for some time after treatment completion, causing false-positive results. The shorter the time period between previous TB and the current episode, the

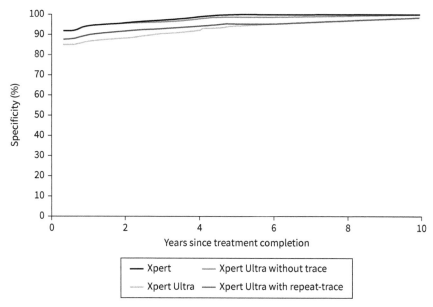

Fig. 3.4 The specificity of Xpert Ultra as a function of time since TB treatment was most recently completed. From Dorman et al. (2018).[3]

more likely it is that remnant DNA will be present. So in order to know the specificity of an individual, it is necessary to know the time since treatment completion.

The take-home message is that sensitivity and specificity are 'unstable' statistics, which can vary widely based on seemingly small differences between studies as well as differences between patients within studies.

The Effect of Prevalence

If you were asked this question in a medical exam 'Does sensitivity vary with disease prevalence?' you might bring up a picture of a 2×2 table in your mind and conclude that sensitivity is based on people who definitely have the disease, this is unrelated to prevalence, and the answer must be 'No'. You would probably get a mark in the exam but in fact the answer is 'Yes'. Mariska Leeflang et al. analysed 416 diagnostic accuracy studies with a range of prevalence from 1% to 77% and found a statistically significant effect of prevalence on both sensitivity and specificity.[4] They conclude that this effect is likely to be the result of mechanisms, such as patient spectrum, that affect prevalence, sensitivity, and specificity. Because it may be difficult to identify such mechanisms, clinicians should use prevalence as a guide when selecting studies that most closely match their situation.

Advanced Knowledge Summary

- Sensitivity and specificity are 'unstable' statistics that can vary widely even when differences between studies seem small.
- Prevalence also affects sensitivity and specificity.

⊙ See Video 3—Sensitivity_and_specificity—available at: https://doi.org/10.1093/med/9780192866615.012.0003.

Notes

1. Ozenne B, Subtil F, Maucort-Boulch D. The precision–recall curve overcame the optimism of the receiver operating characteristic curve in rare diseases. J Clin Epidemiol. 2015;68(8):855–859.
2. Horne DJ, Kohli M, Zifodya JS, Schiller I, Dendukuri N, Tollefson D, et al. Xpert MTB/RIF and Xpert MTB/RIF Ultra for pulmonary tuberculosis and rifampicin resistance in adults. Cochrane Database Syst Rev. 2019;6(6):CD009593.
3. Dorman SE, Schumacher SG, Alland D, Nabeta P, Armstrong DT, King B, et al. Xpert MTB/RIF Ultra for detection of Mycobacterium tuberculosis and rifampicin resistance: a prospective multicentre diagnostic accuracy study. Lancet Infect Dis. 2018;18(1):76–84. Erratum in: Lancet Infect Dis. 2018;18(4):376.
4. Leeflang MM, Rutjes AW, Reitsma JB, Hooft L, Bossuyt PM. Variation of a test's sensitivity and specificity with disease prevalence. CMAJ. 2013;185(11):E537–E544.

4

Test Accuracy As Positive and Negative Predictive Values

In Chapter 3 we saw some of the drawbacks of describing a test in terms of its sensitivity and specificity, the principal one being that these answer questions we rarely if ever ask, such as 'In this patient who definitely has cancer, what is the chance that the test is positive?' We learned that we rarely if ever know which **column** of the 2×2 table a patient belongs in, but when we have a test result we know which **row** they are in. The obvious progression is therefore to look at statistics concerned with **rows** rather than **columns**.

Positive and negative predictive values are exactly that.

Positive predictive value (PPV) answers the question 'In patients with a **positive test**, what is the chance that they **have the condition?**'

It is calculated using only the first row of the 2×2 table as A/(A+B) (Table 4.1).

Negative predictive value (NPV) answers the question 'In patients with a **negative test**, what is the chance that they **do not have the condition?**'

It is calculated using only the second row of the 2×2 table as D/(C+D) (Table 4.2).

This seems to solve the major problem we have with sensitivity and specificity. **Predictive values answer patient-relevant questions.** So what's the catch?

Suppose you want to test a patient for a condition. There are two almost identical diagnostic accuracy studies of the test which give identical sensitivity and specificity values (DAS1 and DAS2) (Table 4.3).

We know that predictive values tell us the probability of a condition being present when a test is positive. If our patient has a positive test and we use DAS1 we get PPV = 198/(198+10) = 95%.

So she is 95% likely to have the condition.

But if we use DAS2 we get PPV = 99/(99+14) = 88%.

So she is 88% likely to have the condition.

This is the same test, performed on the same person, and yet we get two different answers depending on which of two (almost) identical accuracy studies we use.

The answer lies in the prevalence of the condition within the population studied in each diagnostic accuracy study. In DAS1 it is 200 of 450 (44%) and in DAS2, 100 of 450 (22%).

Table 4.1 PPV is concerned only with patients who have a positive test, the first row of a 2×2 table

	Definitely has the condition	Definitely does not have the condition
Test is positive	A	B
Test is negative	C	D

Table 4.2 NPV is concerned only with patients who have a negative test, the second row of a 2×2 table

	Definitely has the condition	Definitely does not have the condition
Test is positive	A	B
Test is negative	C	D

Table 4.3 The results of two theoretical diagnostic accuracy studies (DAS1 and DAS2) of the same test on similar populations. The sensitivity is 99% and specificity 96% in both studies

(a) DAS1

	Definitely has the condition	Definitely does not have the condition
Test is positive	198	10
Test is negative	2	240

Sensitivity = 198/(198+2) = 99%. Specificity = 240/(240+10) = 96%.

(b) DAS2

	Definitely has the condition	Definitely does not have the condition
Test is positive	99	14
Test is negative	1	336

Sensitivity = 99/(99+1) = 99%. Specificity = 335/(336+14) = 96%.

Positive and Negative Predictive Values Vary Depending on the Prevalence of the Condition in the Population That Is Tested

Fig. 4.1 shows how PPV and NPV vary with prevalence when sensitivity is 99% and specificity 96%. On the left, where prevalence is 0% any test will have a PPV of 0% and NPV of 100%, with the reverse being true at 100% prevalence. Between those extremes, predictive values vary with prevalence. The vertical lines represent the prevalence of 22% and 44% and intersect with the PPV line at 88% and 95%, respectively.

It follows from the above that quoting a predictive value without stating the prevalence is meaningless. So, whenever you hear someone say, for example, the PPV is X%, without also saying when the prevalence is Y%, it is a meaningless statement. Feel free to (politely) ask them the prevalence—if they do not know or do not think it is important, perhaps offer them a copy of this book.

A real-life example is rapid point-of-care tests for COVID-19 based on the detection of viral antigens using lateral flow assays. A 2021 review by the Cochrane COVID-19 Diagnostic Test Accuracy Group found that the best performing test is SD Biosensor STANDARD Q with sensitivity of 88.1% and specificity of 99.6% when testing symptomatic people. They quote PPVs in the range of 84–90% at 5% prevalence, which means that between 1 in 10 and 1 in 6 positive results will be a false

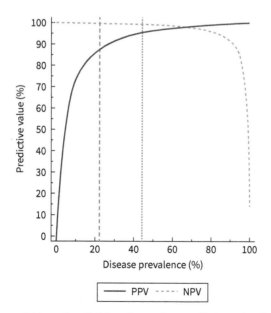

Fig. 4.1 Positive predictive value (PPV) and negative predictive value (NPV) as a function of disease prevalence for a test with sensitivity of 99% and specificity of 96%. First vertical line indicates disease prevalence in DAS2 (22%) and second vertical line DAS1 (44%). Drawn with MedCalc.

positive, and between 1 in 4 and 1 in 8 cases will be missed (false negative). At 0.5% prevalence, applying the same test in asymptomatic people would result in PPVs of only 11–28% meaning that between 7 in 10 and 9 in 10 positive results will be false positives, and between 1 in 2 and 1 in 3 cases will be missed. This is an excellent example of how to appropriately present predictive values and an important lesson in how poor they can be when prevalence is very low, even when the values for sensitivity and specificity look convincing.

So should we abandon predictive values as useless? Absolutely not.

How to Use Predictive Values

Predictive values have the drawback of being influenced by prevalence but in general are much more intuitively useful metrics than sensitivity and specificity. It is vital that predictive values are **always** quoted along with the prevalence in the population from which they are derived. For example, the PPV of anti-double-stranded DNA for lupus is 95% when the prevalence of lupus is 50% in the population you are sampling (perhaps patients with a rash attending a rheumatology clinic) is an intuitively helpful statistic. It at least gives us a better feel for the test than its sensitivity and specificity.

When confronted with an individual, a predictive value will also be useful if the prevalence (strictly pre-test probability which we will encounter in Chapter 4) is the same or similar to the prevalence in which the accuracy study was performed. In the example above, if the prevalence of cancer is around 22% in the population from which the patient is drawn, the PPV of 88% will be fairly accurate for that patient, and answer the patient-relevant question of the probability of cancer.

It must be remembered that predictive values are drawn directly from 2×2 tables and have the same limitations as sensitivity and specificity based on the conduct of the accuracy study.

Summary

- Predictive values answer patient-relevant questions about the probability of disease with a given result.
- Predictive values for the same test vary with disease prevalence.
- Predictive values must **always** be quoted with the disease prevalence.
- Predictive values, when quoted with prevalence, are intuitively more useful than sensitivity and specificity.
- Predictive values are most useful when prevalence in the population from which the person being tested is similar to the prevalence in the population used for the accuracy study.

⊙ See Video 4—Predictive_values—available at:
    https://doi.org/10.1093/med/9780192866615.012.0004.

5
Test Accuracy As Likelihood Ratios

In Chapter 3 we learnt the drawbacks of sensitivity and specificity and in Chapter 4 we learnt that predictive values, when quoted with prevalence, are an improvement. However, predictive values are dependent on prevalence and may not be directly applicable to a patient in front of us. In this chapter we turn to likelihood ratios and Bayes' theorem as a way to circumvent these problems.

What Is Bayes' Theorem?

The history of Bayes' theorem, while fascinating, is not core knowledge, and can be found in Appendix 1 along with a popular example known as the Monty Hall problem. It sounds complex and scary but really isn't.

As it applies to medical tests, Bayes' theorem can be simply described as:

> **Updating the probability of a condition based on a test result.**

Key assumption: we are discussing the diagnosis of a binary (present or absent) condition. In other words, you begin with a probability of the condition being present (**pre-test probability**) then update to a new probability (**post-test probability**). The difference between pre- and post-test probabilities are determined by **properties of the test.**

The **properties of the test** we are interested in are called **likelihood ratios.** When a test is positive, the likelihood ratio is positive (LR+ve) and vice versa (LR−ve). At this point it is fine to consider likelihood ratios as properties of a test calculated from the 2×2 table. The details, which are not vital at this stage, are in Box 5.1.

- LR+ve lies between 1 and infinity—the higher the value, the greater the increase in probability when the test is positive.
- LR−ve lies between 0 and 1—the lower the value, the greater the decrease in probability with a negative test.
- A LR+ve or LR−ve of 1 means that the test result is random and has no effect on the probability of the condition.

Box 5.1 The definitions of LR+ve and LR−ve

LR+ve: the ratio of sick people with a positive test to not sick people with a positive test = sensitivity/(1 − specificity) = (A/(A+C))/(1−D/(B+D)).

LR−ve: the ratio of sick people with a negative test to not sick people with a negative test = (1 − sensitivity)/specificity = (1−A/(A+C))/(D/(B+D)).

Note that a test with a binary outcome will have a LR+ve and a LR−ve. These are not reciprocals of one another but depend on the values in the 2×2 table.

So in order to apply Bayes' theorem, we need a way to calculate the **pre-test probability** and a way to convert it to a **post-test probability** using the **likelihood ratios**.

Calculating Pre-Test Probability

Estimating pre-test probability is often done intuitively by experienced clinicians, but more formal approaches are available. There are no formal methods for calculating the pre-test probability of pregnancy but consider these two women who visit their GP wondering if they might be pregnant and try to estimate it in your own mind.

Fatima is aged 25 and has a 2-year-old child; she has had normal periods since age 14, is having sex regularly with her husband without any contraception, and the first day of her last period was 2 months ago.

Julie is 46 years old; she has never been pregnant despite having regular sex with her husband and never using any form of contraception. She last menstruated 6 months ago but has had no change in weight or abdominal swelling.

As a non-expert, my reasoning for calculating the pre-test probability of pregnancy would go something like this. The chance of an unselected female visiting a GP being pregnant is around 2%, Fatima's age is compatible with high fertility, and she has a previous pregnancy, regular sex with a man without contraception, and a last menstrual period 2 months ago. Each fact increases the probability and I end up estimating 50%.

I also start at 2% for Julie but increase less as her age is 46, perhaps decrease a little because of no previous pregnancies, and increase because of regular intercourse and amenorrhoea. In the end I come up with 10%.

Just like mathematical models, these estimates are undoubtedly wrong but probably useful. An experienced GP would undoubtedly do better than me but it gives you an idea of how you might construct a pre-test probability when no other method is available.

Sometimes we have helpful guides. For example, the probability of Down syndrome in a child can be estimated with a fair degree of accuracy simply by knowing the age of the pregnant woman (Table 5.1).

Other well-known examples include the Wells criteria for pre-test probability of pulmonary embolus (Table 5.2).

Table 5.1 Approximate odds of Down syndrome based on maternal age

Maternal age (years)	Odds of Down syndrome
20	1 in 1667
25	1 in 1250
30	1 in 952
35	1 in 385
40	1 in 106
45	1 in 30
49	1 in 11

Table 5.2 Wells criteria for determining the pre-test probability of pulmonary embolus

Criteria	Points	
Suspected deep vein thrombosis	3	
Alternative diagnosis less likely than pulmonary embolus	3	
Heart rate >100 beats per minute	1.5	
Immobilization/surgery previous 4/52	1.5	
Previous deep vein thrombosis/pulmonary embolus	1.5	
Haemoptysis	1	
Malignancy (active within 6 months)	1	
Risk	**Points**	**Probability of PE (%)**
Low	0–2	3.6
Moderate	3–6	20.5
High	>6	66.7

In recent years, there has been an explosion in risk prediction models that can help with estimating pre-test probability; we will discuss this further in Chapter 6. However, most of the time you will need to rely on a degree of experience and intuition to determine the pre-test probability.

Updating Pre-Test Probability

The simplest way to update pre-test probability with a likelihood ratio is with a web-based calculator[*] or smartphone app[†]. There are many examples where you simply plug in two numbers and the calculation is done for you. As an example, if you plug pre-test probability 10% and LR+ve 25 into an app you will find that post-test probability is around 74%. For anyone interested in the mathematics behind this, I have put a brief summary in Appendix 2, but it is not vital to know.

Before smartphones, the Fagan nomogram[1] was a practical method for calculating post-test probability from pre-test probability and likelihood ratios. It is now obsolete for that purpose but is helpful in understanding the subtleties of Bayes' theorem in this context. It is used by drawing a straight line from the pre-test probability on the left, through the likelihood ratio in the centre, to give the post-test probability on the right (Fig. 5.1). The diagonal line begins at 10%, travels through 25, and intersects at 74%.

There is nothing intuitive about converting 10% to 74% using the factor 25, which is why a smartphone app is useful. Look closely at the left- and right-hand scales of probability and you will notice that they are not evenly spaced. The values are closer together around 50% and more widely spaced at the extremes. This illustrates a vitally important feature of Bayes' theorem, which is that it is much 'harder' to shift probability at the extremes compared to the mid-point. Nor is the effect of likelihood ratios on pre-test probabilities linear. A likelihood ratio of 100 does not increase the pre-test probability ten times more than does a ratio of 10.

The example above is in fact the result of Julie's positive pregnancy test—you can see that the probability increases from 10% to 74% (64% point increase). Fig. 5.2 shows the Fagan nomogram for Fatima.

Using the same test the post-test probability is 96%, an increase of only 46% points. As you can see by looking at the scales, it gets very difficult to increase (or decrease) probability when near the extremes.

An alternative to the Fagan nomogram is a leaf plot[2] (Fig. 5.3). The pre-test probability runs along the diagonal from bottom left (0%) to top right (100%); to determine the post-test probability, follow a vertical line from the pre-test probability to the bowed line, upwards if positive and vice versa, then read off the probability on the

[*] My preferred web-based calculator can be found at: http://araw.mede.uic.edu/cgi-bin/testcalc.pl
[†] Examples include: https://apps.apple.com/za/app/bayes-theorem-calculator/id1501762787 and https://apkcombo.com/bayes-theorem-calculator/com.hiox.BaTemCalcul/

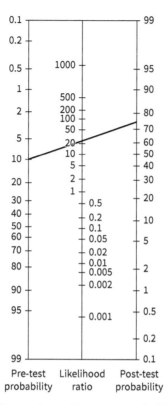

Fig. 5.1 Fagan nomogram for a patient with pre-test probability 10% (left scale) and a positive test with LR+ve 25 (centre scale) showing a post-test probability of 74% (right scale).

vertical axis. The degree of bowing above and below the diagonal correlates with LR+ve and LR−ve respectively. The leaf plot has the disadvantage that it only applies to a single test and must be re-drawn as likelihood ratios change, but an advantage is that it clearly shows how tests change probabilities much more at intermediate pre-test probabilities and much less at the extremes.

When using tests in sequence, the post-test probability of the first test becomes the pre-test probability for the next one. Tests can build on each other in sequence.

The Trouble With Pre-Test Probabilities and Likelihood Ratios

We now seem to have solved the problem of answering the patient relevant question 'What is the probability of the condition being present?' based on the pre-test probability and the diagnostic accuracy of the test. However, this method has limitations.

42

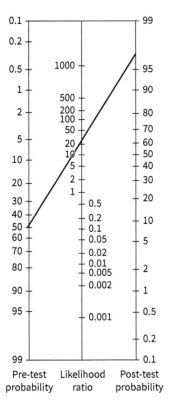

Fig. 5.2 Fagan nomogram for a patient with pre-test probability 50% (left scale) and a positive test with LR+ve 25 (centre scale) showing a post-test probability of 96% (right scale).

It must be remembered that likelihood ratios are calculated directly from 2×2 tables and are therefore susceptible to the same biases as sensitivity and specificity. A likelihood ratio will only be valid if it is calculated from a study of patients similar to the individual in front of you.

As with sensitivity, specificity, and predictive values, likelihood ratios have a margin of error, usually signified by 95% confidence intervals. For tests with several categories of results, extreme test values yield imprecise likelihood ratios. Imprecision in likelihood ratios is greatest at the top and bottom of test result distributions as fewer patients having values that are either very high or low result in little precision. Small changes in the numbers of patients in these cells can produce very different likelihood ratios. Combining continuous categories at the extremes of the test result distribution provides larger numbers and more precision—that is, narrower confidence intervals. Conversely, many test results will fall towards the centre of the distribution. Here, likelihood ratios are closer to 1 and thus help little. The big payoffs stem from high or low likelihood ratios.

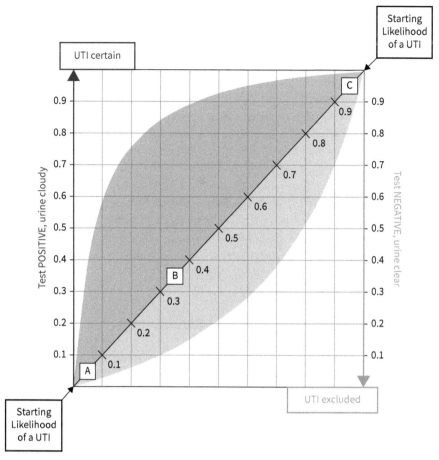

Fig. 5.3 Leaf plot to see how useful it would be to check for urine cloudiness to help diagnose a child's urinary tract infection (UTI), assuming that the test has a sensitivity of 0.75 and specificity of 0.94. The initial estimated probability of the diagnosis of UTI can be anywhere on the diagonal black line from 0 at the bottom left to 1 at the top right, depending on the clinical details. The impact of a positive test (a cloudy urine) is shown by the upwards arrow on the left and shaded area, and is easy to read from the left-hand axis, and the impact of a negative test (a clear urine) is shown by the downwards arrow and shaded area on the right. From Coulthard and Coulthard (2019).[2]

What Is a 'Good' Likelihood Ratio?

It is frequently stated that LR+ve >10 means that a positive test is good at ruling in a diagnosis and a LR−ve <0.1 means that a negative test is good at ruling out a diagnosis. I think by now you will understand how imprecise that statement is. Not only are the results of tests highly context dependent but a likelihood ratio changes the probability by different amounts depending on the starting point.

Imagine a test for Ebola virus with a LR+ve of 10 and LR−ve of 0.1 and to make things as easy as possible for the test, a pre-test probability of 50%. If positive, the post-test probability is 91%; if negative, 9%. During an Ebola outbreak in a low-resource setting, positive patients are cohorted (grouped together without additional infection control between patients). Negative patients are admitted to general hospital wards without specific infection control measures. If you relied on this test with 'good' likelihood ratios, 9% of patients with a positive test would not have Ebola but be sent into a cohort where they would surely contract Ebola virus, and 9% of patients with a negative test would have Ebola and be sent to a general ward where many other patients and staff would undoubtedly become infected. Clearly such a test would not be adequate in these circumstances. In the absence of a more accurate rapid test, the real-world solution is to employ a rapid screening tool (using questions and measuring temperature) that has very high sensitivity (high NPV, low LR−ve) to effectively exclude Ebola from a proportion of patients who are sent to the general wards. The remainders then have to be kept in individual isolation until the results of blood PCR tests are available.

The Example of Prostate Cancer Screening

Screening programmes are typically targeted at populations, but we must still interpret the results of screening tests in individual patients in front of us. We tend to screen large numbers of people to find relatively few cases and so a commonality is that the pre-test probability is very low, which is an important factor in choosing a test. Prostate cancer is the fifth leading cause of male cancer-related deaths worldwide, with around 1.25 million new cases and 350,000 deaths annually. We will take the example of screening for prostate cancer with prostate-specific antigen (PSA) as this has been well studied but remains controversial. PSA is a protein produced by normal prostate glands, its function is to prevent semen from coagulating and it can be detected in blood; levels tend to rise if the prostate becomes cancerous.

PSA results are continuous, with values from zero to >10,000 but most commonly results lie in the range from 1 to 10. Results are commonly dichotomized with a cut-off value of 4.

Let's look at a typical sample of asymptomatic men aged 50–60 who are invited for screening. Published data confirm that the pre-test probability is around 0.1% (1 in 1000). The likelihood ratios of PSA testing have been determined in numerous studies; the typical reference standard being a combination of biopsy of the prostate and in those not undergoing biopsy for ethical reasons, 'being free of cancer' after a period of time. Based on these reference standards and using a PSA break point of 4 (>4 is positive, ≤4 is negative), published LR+ve = 5.5 and LR−ve = 0.61.

The Fagan nomogram (Fig. 5.4) shows us that the post-test probability after a positive test is 0.5%. This minor change is a factor of the pre-test probability being very

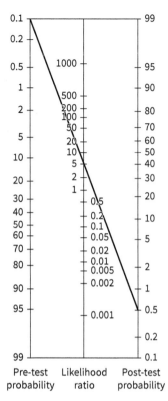

Fig. 5.4 Fagan nomogram for a patient with pre-test probability 0.1% (left scale) and a positive test with LR+ve 5.5 (centre scale) showing a post-test probability of 0.5% (right scale).

low, and the LR+ve not being very high. The post-test probability after a negative test is 0.06%.

In a typical screening programme, men with a negative test would be reassured that they don't have prostate cancer and those with a positive test would be invited for a prostate biopsy. This is done by passing a needle through the rectum into the gland, which as you might imagine is invasive and comes with real risks of bleeding and infection.

Let's follow through what happens if we screen 10,000 men aged 50–60 with a PSA test. The pre-test probability is 1 in 1000 so 10 men will have cancer. Around 800 PSA tests will be positive leading to 800 biopsies; 9200 tests will be negative and these men will be reassured.

Now look at the distribution of cancer among those men. The post-test probability of 0.5% means that four of 800 men with positive tests have cancer, which leaves six men with cancer in the negative test group (approximately 0.06% of 9200).

In summary, if we screen this population we will perform 10,000 blood tests and 800 biopsies, to detect four cancers and we will falsely reassure six men (Fig. 5.5).

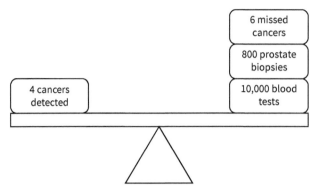

Fig. 5.5 Scales showing the outcome of screening 10,000 men aged 50–60 for prostate cancer using PSA.

Factor in the psychological costs of telling 800 men that their 'cancer test' was positive and you can see why prostate cancer screening with PSA is controversial.

The fundamental problem here is that, as with most screening, the odds are stacked against the test from the beginning because pre-test probability is so low, and we know that tests perform less well at the extremes. A second problem is that the PSA test just isn't that good, LR+ve = 5.5 and LR–ve= 0.61 just isn't up to the job. There is no bigger critic of this form of prostate cancer screening than Dr Richard J. Ablin who discovered PSA in 1970 and has described its use as a screening tool as a 'public health disaster'. The motivation for this is open for debate but Dr Ablin suggests that one reason is the amount of revenue provided for healthcare practitioners and drug companies. The annual bill for prostate cancer screening in the US alone is at least $3 billion.

So what might we do to improve the performance of prostate cancer screening? The obvious answer is to improve the diagnostic accuracy of the test, and the simplest way to do this is by combining PSA testing with a digital rectal examination of the prostate. Other, more exciting possibilities are tests for targets other than PSA which might turn out to be intrinsically more accurate. For example, a test, or combination of tests with LR+ve 10 and LR–ve 0.25, would find 8 of the 10 cancers with only 776 biopsies.

Another option is to increase the pre-test probability by beginning screening at an older age or by taking into account other risk factors such as family history and race (for reasons that aren't well understood, black men have a higher risk of developing and dying of prostate cancer). Increasing pre-test probability to 0.5%, but using the same test would pick up 22 of the 50 cancers with 815 biopsies but 28 of 9185 men would be falsely reassured.

As a result of the poor performance of tests, prostate cancer screening remains controversial; as an example, the US Preventive Services Task Force currently recommends:

- In men aged 55–69 years, the decision to undergo periodic PSA screening should be an individual one after thorough upfront discussion between the physician and patient regarding risks, benefits, and limitations of such screening incorporating the patient's values and preferences in decision-making.

- It recommends against PSA screening in men aged ≥70 years as it offers minimal survival benefit, which does not outweigh the significant treatment side effects and morbidities.

PSA is far from the only screening test to fail to live up to expectations. A recent study screening women for ovarian cancer over 20 years using the blood-based marker cancer antigen (CA)-125 and ultrasound failed to show any benefit in terms of reduced ovarian cancer morbidity and mortality.

Non-Binary Conditions

Up to now we have only considered conditions that are either present or absent such as pregnancy, TB, and appendicitis. However, not all conditions are as clear cut, and as anyone who has read a laboratory report for a haematology or biochemistry test will tell you, many results are presented with reference ranges of some kind. Some laboratory information systems highlight values outside the range in bold or red font. Reference ranges, which are a particular type of reference standard, can have lower or upper boundaries but most commonly have both, and before attempting to interpret them it is important to understand how they are calculated.

Laboratory scientists go to great lengths to provide us with useful reference values and it is not easy. A basic method might be to select a large group of 'healthy people', measure the analyte in question, and plot the results; assuming a normal distribution, the reference range might be quoted as two standard deviations either side of the mean. The difficulties and limitations of such a method are clear: you first need to define 'healthy people', then use exactly the same specimen collection and laboratory methods as the real-world setting. The reference range would then only apply to people within the domain of 'healthy people' you chose, a group with different biological sex, ethnicity, age, and so on might produce different values. Even then you would be left with a reference range where 5% of 'healthy people', by having values greater than two standard deviations from the mean, had an 'abnormal' value; based on this alone you might expect 1 in 20 of all tests on a perfectly healthy person to fall outside the reference range.

The typical reference range for serum sodium is 135–145 mmol/L, and while we could define hyponatraemia as serum sodium <135 mmol/L and accept this as imperfect, it is important to recognize that it is a continuous condition. A value of 134 mmol/L would satisfy the definition but hardly ever requires an intervention, whereas a value of 100 mmol/L indicates a life-threatening condition requiring urgent action. The degree of deviation from the normal range can be captured with categories—such as mild, 130–134 mmol/L; moderate, 125–129 mmol/L; and profound, <125 mmol/L—or by statistics such as Z-scores which indicate the degree of deviation from the mean of 'normal' values.

Reference ranges are challenging to develop and must be used with caution by the clinician. Not only can values outside the reference range be normal, due to the two standard deviation rule, or of minimal importance (serum sodium 134 mmol/L), values within the reference range can also be abnormal. This might be simply because the patient is drawn from a different population than that used to develop the reference range in terms of factors such as age or ethnicity or because the reference range doesn't apply to them as an individual. Take the example of parathyroid hormone (PTH) which is secreted by the parathyroid glands and regulates the serum calcium concentration through its effects on bone, kidney, and intestine. A typical reference range is 14–65 pg/mL but it would be a mistake to interpret a value within that range as normal without also considering the calcium concentration. PTH and calcium are in a feedback loop—when calcium is high it normally suppresses PTH secretion and vice versa, so a patient with abnormally high calcium should have a low PTH. The finding of 'normal' PTH levels in a patient with high calcium is therefore 'abnormal' for that patient, something that would typically be seen in primary hyperparathyroidism. One might say that the PTH level is 'out of keeping' with the calcium level.

Summary

- Bayes' theorem describes the process of updating the probability of a condition being present based on test results (and isn't scary).
- Before a test is done, we calculate the pre-test probability using intuition and experience or, where available, a data-driven approach.
- Likelihood ratios are a property of tests derived from 2×2 tables.
- Pre-test probabilities are combined with likelihood ratios to give post-test probabilities, this is best done with a smartphone app.
- For a given likelihood ratio, probabilities move more around 50% and less at the extremes.
- Screening is typically performed when pre-test probability is low meaning that tests with high diagnostic accuracy are needed.
- We should be cautious in using reference ranges to guide our actions. Values outside the range can require no action and vice versa.

See Video 5—Bayes_theorem—available at: https://doi.org/10.1093/med/9780192866615.012.0005.

Notes

1. Fagan TJ. Letter: Nomogram for Bayes theorem. N Engl J Med. 1975;293(5):257.
2. Coulthard MG, Coulthard T. The leaf plot: a novel way of presenting the value of tests. Br J Gen Pract. 2019;69(681):205–206.

6
Decision Thresholds

Up to this point, we have learnt that tests of individuals can be described by their sensitivity, specificity, predictive values, and likelihood ratios. The latter are the most useful and when combined with pre-test probability, can answer patient-relevant questions such as 'What is the probability of a condition being present in this individual?'

We now turn to the question of whether tests are worth doing. It is very rare for a test to have both LR+ve and LR−ve equal to 1 and so almost all tests change the probability of a condition either up or down, even if not by very much. Put another way, almost all tests add **something** to a clinician's diagnostic reasoning, the question is whether that **something** is of practical value.

A helpful place to begin is with diagnostic and treatment thresholds, which were first introduced in 1975 in a seminal work by Pauker and Kassirer.[1] They realized that in the face of diagnostic uncertainty, clinicians are commonly faced with a dilemma of whether or not to treat a condition. It is that moment when the professor stands at the end of the bed and strokes his beard mindfully before deciding on a course of action. They called this point of equipoise, or indifference, where the decision to treat or not treat is finely balanced the **therapeutic threshold**. It is expressed as a probability of a condition being present above which we should treat, and below which we should not. In plain terms, the therapeutic threshold is the probability above which it is beneficial to intervene, and below which intervention will cause more harm than good.

Key assumptions:

- Only one condition is being considered.
- A well-defined and beneficial treatment is available.
- There is uncertainty about the presence or absence of the condition.
- A patient with the condition who does not receive the treatment undergoes some loss.
- A patient who does not have the disease but nevertheless undergoes the treatment is subject to a finite cost.
- No further investigations are available.
- Resources are plentiful.[*]
- The patient is happy to follow the advice of the clinician.[1]

---

[*] Not included in the original paper but added by the author.

Table 6.1 A 2×2 table regarding the decision to perform or withhold surgery on a patient who may or may not have appendicitis

	Appendicitis	No appendicitis
Surgery	Treat disease (good)	Treat no disease (bad)
No surgery	No treatment of disease (bad)	No treatment no disease (good)

They argued that the therapeutic threshold could be calculated for any condition fulfilling these assumptions so long as costs and benefits could be estimated. They took the example of a patient with right iliac fossa pain in whom there was uncertainty as to whether appendicitis was present. To fulfil the assumptions, they assumed that an alternative cause for right iliac fossa pain was viral gastroenteritis, that surgery was known to be beneficial if appendicitis was present (this was before trials showing that appendicitis can be treated with antibiotics alone in some cases), that a patient with appendicitis who does not have surgery will undergo a cost (perhaps ruptured appendix), and that one with viral gastroenteritis who undergoes surgery with incur a cost (surgical complications).

This can also be viewed as a 2×2 table (Table 6.1).

The beneficial outcomes are treating disease and not treating no disease, the costly outcomes are the opposite.

They ascribed values of 0.1% to operative mortality and 1% to mortality of appendicitis not treated with surgery. When working through the mathematics (see Appendix 3, pun intended) it turns out that the therapeutic threshold is 10%, which means that in order to minimize mortality, if the surgeon thinks the probability of appendicitis is >10% she should operate, and vice versa.

Factors Influencing Treatment Thresholds

The appendicitis example is simplified for the sake of explanation and only takes account of the risks of mortality. In practice, there are a whole range of factors to consider when determining treatment thresholds.

Morbidity

When making a treatment decision we would also consider short- and long-term morbidity. For appendicitis that might be pain or adhesions following ruptured appendix. In other conditions it might include drug side effects and patient anxiety.

Clinical Status

An important consideration that impacts both morbidity and mortality is the clinical status of the patient. The consequences of withholding treatment from a patient who is seriously ill are greater than in a less unwell patient, where there may be time to adjust the decision if necessary.

As an example, consider two patients with community-acquired pneumonia (CAP). Mr Johnson is extremely unwell and likely to need treatment in the intensive care unit while Mr Symcox is less unwell and may need a day or two in hospital at most. Consider that there are three possible aetiologies in both patients: based on clinical evaluation and the epidemiology of infections at the time (e.g. proximity to influenza season and *Mycoplasma* outbreaks), these are considered to be *Streptococcus pneumoniae* (50%), *Mycoplasma pneumoniae* (25%), and influenza virus (25%). There is no rapid and reliable testing available. For simplicity, assume there are three mutually exclusive treatments (each treatment is effective for one pathogen but not the other two). In this situation there are three treatment decisions to make, that is, treat or not treat for each pathogen.

Because Mr Johnson is so sick, the therapeutic thresholds for each one may be <25% so we would give all three drugs, even though we're pretty sure he only has one pathogen. For Mr Symcox, the therapeutic threshold might be >25% but <50% in which case we would treat only for *S. pneumoniae* to begin with, and withhold the other two treatments.

In Mr Johnson's case, if we withhold treatment for *Mycoplasma* and influenza but one of these is the culprit, he may not survive long enough for us to change tack. In Mr Symcox's case, we have time on our side and can safely avoid the possible side effects of these two treatments and see how he responds.

A basic rule of thumb, when the diagnosis is uncertain, is that the more unwell a patient is, the more empiric therapies are necessary. In my own practice, a critically ill patient with advanced HIV and bilateral infiltrates on chest X-ray (CXR), during the influenza season, might be treated for TB, CAP, influenza, COVID-19, and *Pneumocystis jirovecii* pneumonia all at the same time until we are able to confidently exclude some of these aetiologies. A stable patient may have no treatment at all while the diagnostic process is performed.

Financial Costs

Every time you request a laboratory or imaging test, you are consuming financial and human resources. In healthcare systems with finite resources, wastefulness means that more important services must be curtailed. It has been estimated that $6.8 billion of medical care in the US involves unnecessary testing and procedures that do not improve patient care and may even harm the patient,[2] so clearly there is plenty of money to be saved by testing appropriately.

Patient Choice

Holistic medicine includes discussion with patients regarding their treatment options and this should always be considered when making a treatment decision. The appendicitis example only considered short-term mortality as if that was the only relevant factor; it is safe to assume that most people would prefer to minimize their risk of dying but in more realistic scenarios patients may have different opinions in similar situations. For example, one patient might be happy to take a short-term risk in the form of an operation to remove a brain tumour for a long-term gain in terms of longevity, another patient may take a different view and prefer not to undergo the surgery but try chemotherapy and/or radiotherapy.

Determining Treatment Thresholds

In the appendicitis example, Pauker and Kassirer were able to draw on published values for mortality in order to calculate the therapeutic threshold. In real-life situations, not only are things far more complicated, but there will be more unknowns. There are a range of empirical methods for determining thresholds (see 'Advanced knowledge') but in the absence of hard data, one way to intuitively estimate a therapeutic threshold is with a thought experiment.

Imagine 100 identical patients with HIV and cough, they are relatively well and you are seeing them in an outpatient clinic. You are concerned that they might have TB but are unsure. As they are identical, there is no rationale for treating them differently, you must either treat all 100 or treat none. Crucially, no further testing is available to you at this time so you have to make a decision. Either treat all or treat none by adopting a wait-and-see approach. If you were told the probability of TB was 90%, you would probably agree to treat all 100. Your reasoning being that the benefits to the 90 in terms of reduced TB morbidity and mortality would outweigh the costs to the 10 in terms of side effects. Now reduce the probability to 80%, then 70% and carry on until you feel uncomfortable treating all the patients. There comes a point where you would switch strategy to not treating all 100 patients, rationalizing that the side effects to patients without TB would outweigh the benefits to patients with TB. In my mind this comes out at around 25% as I feel comfortable that I could pick up TB in that 25% by waiting and seeing, and perhaps giving treatments for alternative causes of cough. I'm fairly comfortable that they wouldn't come to too much harm or infect too many others during that time. This is balanced against the side effects of treating 75 patients with 6 months of chemotherapy for an illness they don't have. The threshold value in your own mind will likely be different to mine and that's fine. Remember, this is a thought experiment and the patients are identical, so no cheating by deciding to treat only a proportion.

Now change the patients' condition to them being unwell enough to require hospital admission with raised respiratory rate and pulse. Run the same thought experiment and see if the point at which you change strategy alters. My own threshold drops to around 10% in this scenario, but again, yours might be different.

In my experience, this thought experiment makes clinicians very anxious; they tend to want to break the rules and to make a bargain. Often, they will only commit to a range of probabilities above which they will treat, and below which not treat. This might be reasonable given that the patient scenario is abstract, but the fact remains that when attending to an individual patient with a single treatment decision to be made, there is a probability at which the clinician is unsure of what to do—this is the **treatment threshold**.

Application to Requesting Tests

You may be wondering what this has to do with requesting tests. The answer is that therapeutic thresholds become very useful when the assumption 'no further testing is available' is replaced with 'a single diagnostic test with imperfect accuracy is available'.

Pauker and Kassirer used this updated set of assumptions in their 1980 paper.[3] The addition of a test changes decision-making from 'treat' or 'don't treat', to 'test and rely on the result', 'treat without testing', or 'don't treat without testing' and introduces two new thresholds.

The **test–treatment threshold** is the probability above which treatment should be started, even if the test is negative (i.e. treat without testing) and the **test threshold** is the probability below which treatment should not be started even if the test is positive (i.e. exclude the diagnosis without doing the test).

The depiction of the test threshold (T_t) and test–treatment threshold (T_{trx}) is shown in Fig. 6.1 as the original diagram from Pauker and Kassirer in 1980. The probability of the condition runs horizontally from 0 to 1.0.

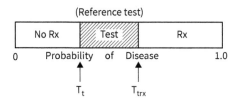

Fig. 6.1 The original diagram depicting test threshold (T_t) and test–treatment threshold (T_{trx}) for a reference test. Disease probability is expressed horizontally from 0 to 1.0 and is divided into areas of no treatment (No Rx), test, and treat (Rx). From Pauker and Kassirer (1980).[3]

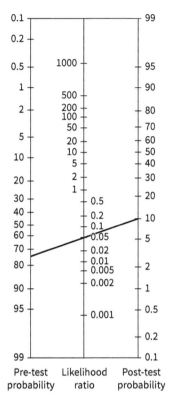

Fig. 6.2 Fagan nomogram showing a test–treatment threshold of 75% (left scale) calculated by the line running from the therapeutic threshold 10% (right scale) through the LR+ve 0.05 (centre scale). Any pre-test probability >75% will produce a post-test probability >10% using the same test and will therefore not influence the decision to offer treatment.

The two thresholds can also be visualized on a Fagan nomogram by moving from right to left; in the appendicitis example, the therapeutic threshold remains at 10% and a test, perhaps an ultrasound scan, with LR−ve 0.05 and LR+ve 10 is available.

In the example in Fig. 6.2, the test–treatment threshold is 75%, defined by the line from 10% (right) through 0.05 (LR−ve). Put another way, for any pre-test probability >75%, a negative test gives a post-test probability >10% and so treatment should be given, **even with a negative test**.

Similarly, the test threshold in the example in Fig. 6.3 is 1%, defined by the line from 10% (right) through 10 (LR+ve). Put another way, for any pre-test probability<1%, a positive test gives a post-test probability <10% and so treatment should not be given, **even with a positive test**.

To summarize, the test–treatment threshold is the pre-test probability above which treatment should be started even if the test is negative and the test threshold is the pre-test probability below which treatment should not be started even if the test is

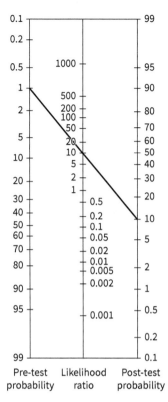

Fig. 6.3 Fagan nomogram showing a test threshold of 1% (left scale) calculated by the line running from the therapeutic threshold 10% (right scale) through the LR+ve 0.05 (centre scale). Any pre-test probability <1% will produce a post-test probability >10% using the same test and will therefore not influence the decision to withhold treatment.

positive, and so in neither case can the test influence the treatment decision. At all other pre-test probabilities, the test should be performed and treatment given according to the result.

It should be clear now that when using tests as diagnostics in similar scenarios they are merely 'tie-breakers'. At the extremes of pre-test probability we don't need tests, or, more accurately, most tests can't help us. This is partly a function of the extended range of probabilities you see at the extremes of the Fagan nomogram. In general, tests aren't good at the extremes and so we shouldn't use them, reserving diagnostic tests for the middle ground when there is genuine indecision. We saw in Chapter 4 that when we attempt to use diagnostic tests at the extremes of pre-test probability in screening programmes, life becomes difficult and we need extremely accurate tests, or more typically combinations of tests in order to improve outcomes.

In the original paper, Pauker and Kassirer calculated the thresholds using values for the costs and benefits of treating and not treating a condition. The possibilities are contained in a 2×4 table (Table 6.2).

Table 6.2 A 2×4 table showing the good and bad outcomes of different combinations of test and treatment decisions based on the presence or absence of a disease

	Disease present	Disease absent
Treat without testing	Good	Bad
Test positive—treat	Good	Bad
Test negative—don't treat	Bad	Good
Don't test and don't treat	Bad	Good

They also included an assumption that the test itself also carried some risk to the patient, which adds to the complexity. The example they used was of a patient with renal dysfunction and hypertension, the diagnostic decision was between steroid-responsive renal disease (vasculitis) and steroid non-responsive renal disease (malignant hypertension). The test was a renal biopsy which carries significant risks of complications. By assigning values to the benefits of treating vasculitis with steroids, the harms of not treating vasculitis with steroids, the harms of treating malignant hypertension with steroids, the risks of the biopsy, and the accuracy of the test, they determined the test threshold to be 7% and the test–treatment threshold to be 32%. In other words, if the probability of vasculitis was <7%, it would be beneficial not to put the patient through a biopsy with the possibility of a false-positive result, but rather to withhold steroids. If the probability was >32%, the risks of the biopsy and a falsely negative result were outweighed by the benefits of steroids and treatment should be started. At any probability from 7% to 32%, the biopsy should be performed and treatment given according to the result.

When tests have minimal side effects and financial costs, both thresholds can be determined from the therapeutic threshold and likelihood ratios using Bayes' theorem, as described above.

More Examples

Below is an example where patient choice has a profound influence on both testing and treatment decisions. Jamila is a 33-year-old with three children who has finished her family and does not want to become pregnant again. Thandi is a 33-year-old with no children; she recently married a man and is keen to start a family. Let's say that they both have an abnormal cervical smear followed by a biopsy which is inconclusive and suggests a 50% chance of cervical cancer. When considering further testing each has a 50% pre-test probability of cancer. For the sake of the example, let's restrict the choice to either having a hysterectomy (removal of the womb) or undergoing more invasive tests to try to confirm the diagnosis.

Each woman may feel differently about this choice. Jamila may feel that a 50% chance of cancer is enough to opt for a hysterectomy, reasoning that she does not want to become pregnant again and would prefer to know that once the hysterectomy is performed, she will no longer be at risk of cervical cancer. Thandi, on the other hand, may see things differently. She probably would not want a hysterectomy unless it was absolutely necessary because she is about to start a family. Obviously, she also would not want cervical cancer so she might opt for more testing. So for Jamila, the test–treatment threshold is <50%, whereas for Thandi it is >50%. This is essentially because the 'risk' to Thandi of a hysterectomy is higher because she wants to have children.

This is an example of the crucial role played by patients' own judgements in making medical decisions. For simplicity, this was excluded from the original Pauker and Kassirer papers but can clearly have a profound effect on the appropriate course of action.

This is a good time to revisit some concepts we met in Chapter 2. You will often hear people say that 'So and so is a good "rule-in" test or a good "rule-out" test' by which they mean high sensitivity and specificity respectively. We previously met the aide-memoire SpIN, which means tests with high Specificity are good at ruling a condition IN and SnOUT, which means tests with high Sensitivity are good at ruling a condition OUT. Now think of these in terms of the treatment threshold. A useful 'rule-in' test will occur when we commonly encounter patients where the pre-test probability is between test and treatment thresholds and a positive test increases that probability above the treatment threshold. A useful 'rule-out' test will occur when we commonly encounter patients where the pre-test probability is between treatment and test treatment thresholds and a negative result decreases probability below the treatment threshold.

A test will only truly be a useful 'rule-in' or 'rule-out' test when these conditions are met. A real example from my own field is diagnosing TB in very sick patients with HIV and a cough who are admitted to hospital. Approximately 50% of these patients have TB and as they are very sick the treatment threshold is <50%, let's say 25%. In this scenario, tests with high specificity and PPV and LR+ve are not particularly useful as they simply increase the probability to >50%. What we require is a test with high sensitivity and NPV and low LR−ve to decrease the probability to <25% such that we can withhold treatment. So in this instance it isn't very helpful for someone to say that they have found a great new 'rule-in' test, what we need are great 'rule-out' tests. This is just one example, there are others, even within the field of TB and HIV where we need great 'rule-in' tests. The point is that when you hear such terms you should critically appraise them to see if they make sense in the given scenario.

Summary

- Almost all tests increase or decrease the probability of a condition, but this may not be clinically useful.
- The treatment threshold is the probability above which treatment should be offered and vice versa when no further tests are available for a single condition.

- Many factors including morbidity, mortality, cost, and patient choice influence the value of the treatment threshold.
- When a single imperfect test is available, the test–treatment threshold is the probability above which treatment would be started even if the test is negative.
- The test threshold is the probability below which treatment would not be started even if the test is positive.
- Both thresholds can be calculated from the treatment threshold and likelihood ratios of the test when direct harm to patients and costs are minimal.

Advanced Knowledge

Many of the key assumptions of the Pauker and Kassirer papers described previously are commonly true. The exception is that 'only one condition is being considered'. The implication being that an alternative cause of the symptoms doesn't require a treatment decision. In the example of appendicitis, the competing diagnosis was viral gastroenteritis which requires supportive therapy similar to a patient with appendicitis and in the vasculitis versus malignant hypertension example the assumption was that the severe hypertension would require treatment in its own right regardless of the diagnosis, so only the question of steroids was relevant. So, while there were competing diagnoses in each example, the alternative diagnoses required no change in therapy.

In real life, however, it is common for competing diagnoses to require different treatments, which complicates matters somewhat.

In much of medicine, Occam's razor or the law of parsimony applies. This essentially translates as 'If the patient has multiple symptoms, it's most likely that a single condition accounts for all of them.'* When the number of possible conditions is also limited, Sherlock Holmes' phrase 'When you have eliminated the impossible, whatever remains, however improbable, must be the truth' is also useful. Put simply, if you are confident that only two diagnoses are possible, reducing the probability of one, increases the probability of the other.

Take the example of a patient with HIV and a CD4 count of 50 cells/mL who presents with 3 weeks of headache and neck stiffness. CSF examination reveals pressure 25 mm/H_2O, 100 lymphocytes/$\times 10^6$/L 10 neutrophils $\times 10^6$/L, protein 1 g/mL, and glucose 2.5 g/dL. For the sake of this example, we will consider cryptococcal meningitis and TB meningitis as the only two possibilities (given the duration of symptoms and CSF results, there are few other possibilities). The key test at this point is a cryptococcal antigen (CrAg) test of the CSF (there are different kinds of tests but they have similar properties). The CrAg test at hand has LR+ve 100 and LR−ve 0.025 in this population. The treatment threshold for cryptococcal meningitis is low,

---

* In advanced HIV disease, and other profound immunodeficiencies, Hickam's dictum 'patients can have as many diseases as they darn well please' is often more appropriate.

balancing 100% morality untreated with significant risks of side effects if treatment is given to patients without the disease. A reasonable first approximation might be 5%. If we assume 50% pre-test probability of each diagnosis, a positive CrAg test increases the probability of cryptococcal meningitis to 99%, definitely above the treatment threshold, and a negative test reduces it to 3%, definitely below the treatment threshold. Given that we are only considering two diagnoses in this example, a negative CrAg test not only reduces the probability of cryptococcal meningitis but also increases the probability of TB meningitis, and vice versa. Therefore, the probability of TB meningitis after a negative CrAg test will be approximately 97%, almost certainly above the test–treatment threshold meaning that no further testing is required.[*]

Methods of Determining Thresholds

Several methods of determining thresholds have been used and can be broadly divided into prescriptive (based on calculations) or descriptive (derived from observing clinical practice). Prescriptive methods can be based purely on values of costs and benefits from the literature (e.g. expected utility theory) as used by Pauker and Kassirer or include subjective values and socioeconomic factors (e.g. regret-based models and dual processing threshold models). Descriptive methods rely on decision-making by clinicians when faced with clinical scenarios (e.g. derived thresholds and discrete choice experiments). All methods have strengths and weaknesses and there is no consensus on the best approach. It may be that the optimal strategy is to combine multiple different methods.

> See Video 6—Clinical_thresholds—available at:
> https://doi.org/10.1093/med/9780192866615.012.0006, and
>
> Video 7—Summary—available at:
> https://doi.org/10.1093/med/9780192866615.012.0007,
> which summarizes Chapters 1–6.

Notes

1. Pauker SG, Kassirer JP. Therapeutic decision making: a cost-benefit analysis. N Engl J Med. 1975;293(5):229–234.
2. Freedman DB. Towards better test utilization—strategies to improve physician ordering and their impact on patient outcomes. *EJIFCC*. 2015;26(1):15–30.
3. Pauker SG, Kassirer JP. The threshold approach to clinical decision making. N Engl J Med. 1980;302(20):1109–1117.

---

[*] Real life is always more complicated as TB meningitis and cryptococcal meningitis coexist in a small proportion of patients.

7
Frameworks for Evaluating Medical Tests

Up to now, we have discussed the evaluation of novel tests and their application to individuals. We are now going to take a step back and consider the introduction of a new test from a public health perspective. When presented with a new test, policymakers need to decide whether to introduce it to a healthcare system. In privately funded healthcare, it might be the insurance company that decides whether or not to pay for the new test. In publicly funded healthcare, a government-appointed body might be responsible for the decision. Decisions are also made at international level; the WHO publishes an essential diagnostics list,[1] which is a basket of *in vitro* diagnostics that it recommends be available at point of care and in laboratories in all countries to increase timely and life-saving diagnoses. While the equivalent list for drugs, the essential drugs list, was first published in 1977, the first essential diagnostics list wasn't published until 2018. In order to make these kinds of decisions, it is vital for policymakers to have a clear understanding of how to appropriately evaluate tests as a public health intervention. In the next three chapters we will consider frameworks for test evaluation, discuss the development of diagnostic strategies, and describe testing these strategies in controlled clinical trials.

The key principle of medical test evaluation is the fundamental premise that its introduction will improve health outcomes, or provide other benefits such as reducing costs, or simplifying healthcare delivery without compromising the well-being of patients. Therefore, evaluation begins with defining the potential health outcomes (benefits and harms) of the test that are most relevant to patients. Since tests usually do not affect health outcomes directly, one has to define, right at the beginning of the evaluation process, the purpose and role of the medical test in the clinical pathway and the relevant patient population for each testing application. Test purpose describes the intended clinical application of the test and how the test information will be used to improve clinical management in practice.

Before considering frameworks for test evaluation, it is worth revisiting the evaluation of novel drugs. After all, although drugs typically have a direct, rather than an indirect health benefit, they have many similarities to tests such as costs to health systems and side effects. New drugs are evaluated in humans with a standard four-phase framework, moving on to the next phase if results are acceptable. Phase I studies safety, tolerability, toxicity, pharmacodynamics, and pharmacokinetics by giving the drug to a small group of healthy volunteers, sometimes in incrementally higher doses. Phase II further assesses safety as well as if a drug works, with small-scale clinical investigations on patients with the target condition. The aim of a phase III trial is to determine the effectiveness of the drug by comparing it to the standard of care, which may be an existing drug or a placebo if there is currently no effective therapy. Typically, this will be a randomized clinical trial enrolling anywhere from a few hundred to a few thousand patients. Regulatory approval usually follows successful phase III clinical trials. Phase IV studies assess drugs after they have been released to the market to determine the long-term effects and rare side effects that may not be adequately detected by phase III trials.

This process has traditionally been considered linear, beginning with cheaper, faster, and less risky phase I studies and moving to the next phase only if there is evidence of safety and/or efficacy. However, it is recognized that drug development is actually a cyclic, repetitive process that begins with the recognition of a problem and continues through an expansive thinking phase to experimentation, assessment, and adoption. This process may be repeated as the technology is improved or modified for new uses. The process also cycles and moves 'up the rungs' from laboratory to applied research and, ultimately, to clinical application, and it sometimes slips back to address unanticipated problems and then advances again as those problems are resolved.

There is currently no standard framework for evaluating medical tests that is analogous to drug development; instead, multiple models have been proposed. Lijmer et al. performed a systematic search of the literature and identified 19 schemes published between 1978 and 2007.[2] One of the best known is the levels of efficacy for imaging tests, proposed by Fryback and Thornbury in 1991.[3] Level 1 concerns technical quality of the images; level 2 addresses diagnostic accuracy, sensitivity, and specificity associated with interpretation of the images. Level 3 focuses on whether the information produces change in the referring physician's diagnostic thinking. Level 4 efficacy concerns the effect on the patient management plan and level 5 efficacy studies measure (or compute) the effect of the information on patient outcomes. Finally, at level 6, analyses examine societal costs and benefits of a diagnostic imaging technology. This approach has been widely accepted but is not necessarily applicable outside of imaging studies.

Another framework proposed by Sackett and Haynes has four phases,[4] framed as questions. Phase I questions ask 'Do test results in patients with the target disorder differ from those in normal people?' Phase II questions ask 'Are patients with certain test results more likely to have the target disorder than patients with other test results?' Phase III questions ask 'Does the test result distinguish patients with and without the target disorder among patients in whom it is clinically reasonable to suspect that the disease is present?' Phase IV questions ask 'Do patients who undergo the test fare better (in their ultimate health outcomes) than similar patients who are not tested?'

Common phases among the 19 frameworks identified by Lijmer et al. were evaluations of technical efficacy, diagnostic accuracy, diagnostic thinking efficacy, therapeutic efficacy, patient outcome, and societal aspects. They similarly argue that evaluation of tests is most likely not a linear but a cyclic and repetitive process. Despite these commonalities, there is no unified and widely accepted framework for evaluating novel tests. It's notable that the WHO essential diagnostics list does not provide a framework, rather it calls a meeting of a Strategic Advisory Group of Experts on *in vitro* diagnostic tests (SAGE IVD) that makes recommendations based on factors that include public health and clinical need, availability of validated commercial tests, clinical utility, diagnostic accuracy, cost-effectiveness, infrastructure requirements, and appropriateness to specified healthcare setting.

Rather than propose a unified framework at this point, and in the interests of simplicity, I would like to simply divide test evaluation into three broad phases. The first is 'test research', which determines diagnostic accuracy and is covered in Chapter 1. Test research actually encompasses the first three phases of the Sackett and Haynes framework. In Chapter 7 we will turn to the second phase, 'diagnostic* research', which draws together as much relevant information about a patient as possible to develop 'diagnostic strategies', often in the form of algorithms or prediction rules. Third, in Chapter 8 we move to 'diagnostic intervention research' which is similar to phase IV of the Sackett and Haynes framework and also encompasses level 6 of the Fryback and Thornbury framework by determining if diagnostic strategies improve real-world outcomes of patients and at what cost.

At this point it is worth reflecting on the processes and costs of regulating new drugs and diagnostics. Before a new drug can be sold, it requires regulatory approval. Each country or region typically has a regulatory body such as the Food and Drug Administration (FDA) in the US and the Medicines and Healthcare products Regulatory Agency (MHRA) in the UK. New drugs typically have to be safe and effective in phase III trials before they receive regulatory approval, although exceptions occur when serious diseases are otherwise untreatable, particularly in outbreak scenarios where time is of the essence. The process of regulatory approval for new drugs is typically in-depth and requires review by a committee to determine that it provides benefits that outweigh its known and potential risks for the intended population. By virtue of requiring phase III trials, the process of approval is time-consuming and expensive. When the whole process from discovery to regulation is considered, the average cost of drug development is around $1.3 billion.[5] The median cost of the clinical trial component is around $19 million. Even so, there is a list of drugs which were withdrawn from the market due to safety concerns, even though they initially received regulatory approval.

The requirements for regulatory approval of new diagnostic tests are much less stringent and more variable between agencies. In the US, for example, diagnostic testing, and interpreting those tests, is considered the practice of medicine and the

---

* While I use the term diagnostic for simplicity, the same principles apply equally to prognostic tests research.

FDA is not allowed to regulate the practice of medicine. Yet it is responsible for regulating medical devices such as machines, sample tubes, and other tools that are clearly medical devices. There is no requirement for anything similar to a phase III drug trial, merely that 'it be concluded by qualified experts that there is reasonable assurance of the safety and effectiveness of a device under its conditions of use'. As a result, a more typical estimate for the average cost of developing and commercializing a diagnostic properly in the US is $50–75 million, with around $2.5–7.5 million being spent on 'clinical utility trials'.[6]

As a result of the difference in regulatory requirements for drugs and tests, it's unheard of for new drugs not to undergo phases III and IV clinical trials, whereas tests often only require basic 'test research' before they enter the market. As a result, 'diagnostic research' and 'diagnostic intervention research' are commonly not performed at all. In my view, this is a great shame. While it can be important to get new tests into healthcare systems quickly, and it may be reasonable to adopt some tests without controlled clinical trials, such trials are unlikely to receive appropriate funding if not demanded by regulators when circumstances allow.

Notes

1. World Health Organization. The Selection and Use of Essential in Vitro Diagnostics. WHO Technical Report Series, No. 1031. Geneva: World Health Organization; 2021. Available at: https://www.who.int/publications/i/item/9789240019102.
2. Lijmer JG, Leeflang M, Bossuyt PM. Proposals for a phased evaluation of medical tests. Med Decis Making. 2009;29(5):E13–E21.
3. Fryback DG, Thornbury JR. The efficacy of diagnostic imaging. Med Decis Making. 1991;11(2):88–94.
4. Sackett DL, Haynes RB. The architecture of diagnostic research. BMJ. 2002;324 (7336):539–541.
5. Wouters OJ, McKee M, Luyten J. Estimated research and development investment needed to bring a new medicine to market, 2009–2018. JAMA. 2020;323(9):844–853.
6. Keeling P. Mystery solved! What is the cost to develop and launch a diagnostic? Diaceutics; 2013. Available at: https://www.diaceutics.com/articles/mystery-solved-what-is-the-cost-to-develop-and-launch-a-diagnostic

8
Diagnostic and Prognostic Research

Diagnostic and prognostic research may be loosely defined as the process of drawing together multiple sources of information about patients to develop diagnostic strategies with the aim of improving outcomes. It acknowledges that single tests are rarely used in isolation, and are typically incorporated into a process for answering patient-relevant questions.

One increasingly popular form of diagnostic and prognostic research is the development of multivariable prediction models (MPMs), also variously called clinical or risk prediction rules or models. Well-known examples include the Framingham Risk Score (FRS), QRISK3, Model for Endstage Liver Disease, and ABCD^2 score. MPMs provide accurate and (internally and externally) validated estimates of probabilities of specific health conditions or outcomes in targeted patients, which guide clinicians' decision-making, and consequently improve individual outcomes and the cost-effectiveness of care.

The process of creating and validating a new MPM is set out in two landmark papers by giants of the field: 'Risk prediction models: I. Development, internal validation, and assessing the incremental value of a new (bio)marker'[1] and 'Risk prediction models: II. External validation, model updating, and impact assessment'[2]. There is also a consensus statement called TRIPOD (Transparent Reporting of a multivariable prediction model for Individual Prognosis Or Diagnosis)[3] which clearly sets out how the development and validation of new MPMs should be reported. There is no substitute for reading these papers yourself although I will summarize them here.

The objective of an MPM is to enable objective estimation of probabilities of a disease being present or the risk of developing a disease according to different combinations of predictor values in study participants. For example, the FRS predicts the 10-year probability of cardiovascular disease occurring in adults, depending on predictors of sex, age, smoking status, total cholesterol, high-density lipoprotein cholesterol, and systolic blood pressure.

To develop an MPM you first need a dataset, which should ideally be collected prospectively from a cohort or participants in a randomized trial. The FRS is developed from data collected in the Framingham Heart Study (FHS), which initiated its first cohort in 1948 and is now enrolling the grandchildren of the original participants. All FHS cohorts have been examined approximately every 2–4 years since the initiation of the study. At these periodic examinations, the investigators obtain a medical history and perform a cardiovascular-focused physical examination, 12-lead electro-cardiogram (ECG), blood and urine testing, and other cardiovascular imaging studies reflecting subclinical disease burden. More recently, samples have been taken to study serum and urine biomarkers, genetics/genomics, proteomics, metabolomics, and social networks.[4] The choice of possible predictors to be collected in a study is not always easy: theoretically, all potential and not necessarily causal factors that correlate with the outcome of interest should be collected but this is often impractical. In practice, predictors are typically chosen based on previous publications showing associations with the outcome of interest.

In the FHS, clinical events (outcomes) such as myocardial infarction, coronary insufficiency, angina, coronary heart disease death, sudden coronary disease death, coronary artery bypass surgery, and percutaneous transluminal coronary angiography are also prospectively collected to complete the dataset.

Once you have a dataset with predictors and outcomes you can develop an MPM for those outcomes. There are whole books written on these methods and this is beyond the scope of this book but a basic method that is often used is regression analysis with backwards selection of candidate predictors.

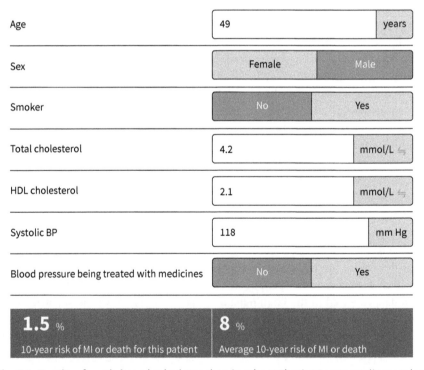

Fig. 8.1 Results of a web-based calculator showing the author's 10-year cardiovascular risk based on data from the FHS. BP, blood pressure; HDL, high-density lipoprotein; MI, myocardial infarction.

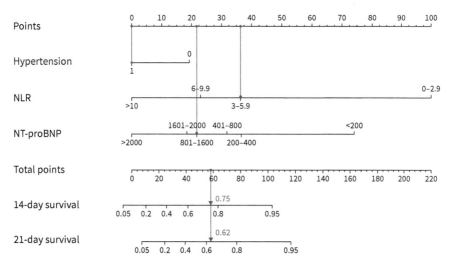

Fig. 8.2 The final nomogram consisting of neutrophil-to-lymphocyte ratio (NLR), hypertension, and N-terminal pro-B-type natriuretic peptide (NT-proBNP) is shown. The usage of the nomogram is illustrated in a hypothetical patient with hypertension, an NLR of 4.0, and NT-proBNP of 1000 pg/mL upon admission (vertical red lines). According to the nomogram, points for hypertension, NLR, and NT-proBNP were 0, 22, and 36, respectively. The total points added up to 58 for this patient, which represented approximately 0.75 and 0.62 of 14- and 21-day in-hospital survival probability (indicated in the nomogram).

Completed models can be presented in a variety of ways. Fig. 8.1 shows my results from a web-based calculator of my 10-year cardiovascular risk based on FHS data. I simply inputted my data and clicked one button.

Models are also sometimes presented as nomograms. Fig. 8.2 is an example from a journal I just happen to be reading today.[5] It predicts the 14-day and 21-day survival of patients with COVID-19 pneumonia.

Models are evaluated for their performance by their discrimination and calibration. Discrimination is the ability of a model to distinguish individuals who experienced the outcome from those who did not. The C-index (equal to the area under the ROC curve (AUC) that we saw in Chapter 3) is the most widely used statistic. Fig. 8.3 shows the ROC and AUC for the nomogram in Fig. 8.2.

Calibration is the agreement between the probability of developing the outcome of interest within a certain time period as **predicted** by the model and the **actual** observed outcome frequencies. It is ideally assessed visually by plotting one against the other graphically and with statistical 'goodness of fit' tests. See Fig. 8.4 for the calibration plots for the nomogram in Fig. 8.2.

Unsurprisingly, models tend to perform particularly well when reapplied to the data from which they were developed, so-called overfitting or optimism. It is therefore

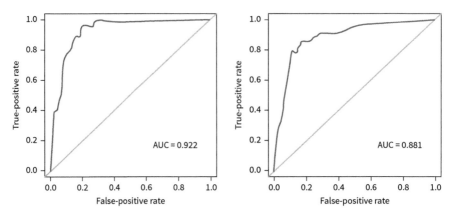

Fig. 8.3 The ROC curve and AUC of the nomogram in the validation cohort. Left and right graphs illustrate 14- and 21-day survival prediction respectively.

important to internally validate (using data from the original dataset) and externally validate (using data from similar but separate datasets) all MPMs.

A common method of internal validation is to randomly divide the dataset into two groups. The first group is usually slightly larger (typically two-thirds of participants) and is used to develop the model. The second, smaller group is used for validation. That is why Fig. 8.3 and Fig. 8.4 refer to the validation cohorts. While this procedure is common, a more complex statistical technique known as bootstrapping is actually preferred as all data are used for both development and validation.

External validation means applying the model to a separate but comparable dataset to determine its performance. The new dataset might be individuals from the same institution in a different, usually later, time period (temporal validation), from a

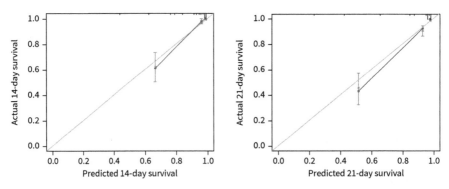

Fig. 8.4 Calibration plot of the nomogram in validation cohorts. Left and right graphs illustrate the calibration plot for predicting 14-day and 21-day survival respectively. Actual rate of survival is shown on the y-axis, and the nomogram-predicted probability of survival is shown on the x-axis.

different location (geographical validation), or from a different domain (domain validation). Different domains might mean, for example, validating a model developed for primary care in patients from secondary care.

Machine Learning Approaches

A new and exciting approach to developing MPM comes from the world of machine learning (ML). ML is essentially the process of computers learning to provide useful outputs without being specifically programmed and is a key part of the so-called fourth industrial revolution. The range of approaches to ML is bewildering and the pace of change rapid; a clinician can't hope to stay up to date with every aspect but it is important to understand the basics as MPMs are increasingly being developed using ML techniques. There is even an update to the TRIPOD statement, called the TRIPOD-Machine Learning statement in development. By the time you read this book, this update will likely be published and easily found with a simple Google search. It aims to focus on the introduction of ML prediction algorithms, building on a long and established methodology of prediction research, while harmonizing terminology.

One important distinction to keep in mind is between tabular and image data. Tabular data is the kind collected in the FHS, essentially rows and columns of numbers signifying each variable. Image data is exactly that, images such as CXRs and ECGs. Techniques you might hear about for developing models from tabular data include random Forest and CART analysis. Interestingly, despite the undoubted potential of ML techniques, results from tabular data have yet to surpass older techniques such as regression.[6]

It is in the analysis of medical images that ML techniques are already flourishing using so-called deep learning methods such as convolutional neural networks. The most established field to date is automated analysis of retinal images to diagnose diabetic retinopathy, but huge progress is currently being made in radiology and other interesting areas such as ECG interpretation.

Notes

1. Moons KG, Kengne AP, Woodward M, Royston P, Vergouwe Y, Altman DG, et al. Risk prediction models: I. Development, internal validation, and assessing the incremental value of a new (bio)marker. Heart. 2012;98(9):683–690.
2. Moons KG, Kengne AP, Grobbee DE, Royston P, Vergouwe Y, Altman DG, et al. Risk prediction models: II. External validation, model updating, and impact assessment. Heart. 2012;98(9):691–698.

3. Collins GS, Reitsma JB, Altman DG, Moons KG. Transparent Reporting of a multivariable prediction model for Individual Prognosis or Diagnosis (TRIPOD): the TRIPOD statement. Ann Intern Med. 2015;162(1):55–63.
4. Tsao CW, Vasan RS. Cohort profile: the Framingham Heart Study (FHS): overview of milestones in cardiovascular epidemiology. Int J Epidemiol. 2015;44(6):1800–1813.
5. Dong YM, Sun J, Li YX, Chen Q, Liu QQ, Sun Z, et al. Development and validation of a nomogram for assessing survival in patients with COVID-19 pneumonia. Clin Infect Dis. 2021;72(4): 652–660.
6. Christodoulou E, Ma J, Collins GS, Steyerberg EW, Verbakel JY, Van Calster B. A systematic review shows no performance benefit of machine learning over logistic regression for clinical prediction models. J Clin Epidemiol. 2019;110:12–22.

9
Impact Studies

Up to this point, we have discussed the initial evaluation of tests in diagnostic accuracy studies and the development of diagnostic and prognostic strategies through diagnostic and prognostic research. We now turn to considering the ultimate goal of tests which is to improve patient outcomes and reduce costs. In this chapter we will use the term test and diagnostic or prognostic strategy interchangeably to acknowledge that intervention research can take different forms. In either case, we will look at studies designed to determine how well these improve patient outcomes and reduce costs, a common name for these are impact studies.

Neither tests nor diagnostic strategies are developed to replace doctors, but to provide **objective** estimates of disease risks or probabilities of current disease and to assist healthcare providers in their **subjective** interpretations, intuitions, and use of guidelines. Their use is also not restricted to healthcare providers and might equally be provided to patients to assist them with self-management decisions. In either case, diagnostic strategies aim to improve patient outcomes and cost-effectiveness of care by providing information that changes individuals' decisions for the better.

There are two main approaches to influencing caregivers' decisions: the assistive approach means providing model outcomes, such as probabilities of a diagnosis in question without recommending decisions. The directive decision approach explicitly recommends or even prescribes specific decisions depending on the probability. The assistive approach is more respectful of the judgement of individuals and doctors and leaves room for intuition, but a decisive approach may have a greater clinical impact. It has been argued that conducting a trial with an assistive rather than a directive approach is like trialling new drugs without prespecifying the preferred dosage, route of administration, need for monitoring, or the way to deal with side effects. The converse is that it might not be appropriate to apply testing strategies without considering factors that were not considered in prior research. In essence, doctors are trained to make sensible decisions when faced with outlying events and it might not make sense to constrain them to rigid rules. In contrast, nurses commonly make important treatment decisions, particularly in low-resource settings, and it might be appropriate to use a more decisive approach with this cadre of healthcare worker.

There are a variety of possible trial designs for impact studies, each with associated costs and benefits. A simple and cheap design may not even include follow-up of patients. For example, we may aim to measure the influence on the behaviour or decision-making of healthcare professionals using a cross-sectional study with decisions as the primary outcome. In this approach, clinicians are randomized to either receiving or not receiving predictions from models or test results and their therapeutic or other management decisions are compared. Even simpler is a before–after study design within the same clinicians. They are asked to make a treatment or management decision for an individual before they have been provided with the individual's predicted risk by the model, and this is compared with the decision they make after they have seen the result. As with phase I or II studies of new drugs, such trial designs are cheap and fast. If they show no impact on behaviour it might be decided not to spend time and money on further evaluation. On the other hand, a positive result does not necessarily equate to improvement in patient outcomes.

When outcomes are relatively rare, or when a long follow-up is required, a cost-effective design may be decision analytic modelling. This approach starts with a well-developed and externally validated model, and combines information on model predictions with information about the effectiveness of treatments from randomized therapeutic trials or meta-analyses. If such an approach fails to show improved outcomes or favourable cost-effectiveness, a more expensive randomized trial may not be attempted.

Other approaches are sometimes used, for example, the prospective 'before–after' impact study. Essentially, outcomes of interest are measured in a time period before and after the diagnostic strategy are introduced. However, this design is sensitive to temporal changes in things like therapeutic approaches and therefore biased results.

The ideal evaluation of a novel diagnostic or prognostic strategy, or test, is in a randomized trial, measuring outcomes that are relevant to patients, such as reduced morbidity and mortality, and relevant to healthcare systems, such as reduced costs. Such trials can be considered akin to phase III clinical trials of new drugs, they are expensive and time-consuming, and as they are not required for test approval, unlike with new drugs, they are often not performed at all.

Randomized comparisons have several advantages over other methods of comparing medical interventions. Random assignment of patients to the strategies under study should prevent any bias in the selection of patients. This basic principle opens up the application of experimental statistical design, such as testing for significance and calculating confidence intervals. Randomized controlled trials are also attractive from a pragmatic point of view: if randomization coincides with a choice between two management strategies, trial design closely mimics existing clinical dilemmas.

Randomized trials are typically conducted by randomly assigning a control group to usual care, while the intervention group is managed according to the strategy in question, using either the assistive or directive approach. Individual randomization, as is typically used in drug trials, where participants seen by a single clinician are randomly assigned to control or intervention groups, is appealing. However, this design can be prone to a learning bias, meaning that the clinician might be influenced to change their management of patients randomized to the control group based on what they have learnt from managing patients in the intervention group. This might reduce the difference between the two groups and cause us to falsely abandon a useful strategy. Imagine, for example, that you are given a new tool for calculating risk of pulmonary embolus based on four clinical features and asked to use it to determine which patients proceed to a definitive CT pulmonary angiogram. After using the tool a few times in intervention patients, you might be able to determine the outcome of the model simply from knowing the inputs. In that situation, you would most likely start to apply that knowledge to control patients, however unconsciously.

As a result of this learning bias, it is more typical to randomize clinicians rather than participants. Often this will be groups from the same centre, known as a cluster, which also helps to reduce learning between clinicians at the same site. This is known as a cluster randomized trial.

An appealing variant of a cluster randomized trial is the stepped-wedge cluster randomized trial meaning that clusters are randomly allocated time periods when they introduce the intervention. All the clusters apply both control and intervention, but the time when they switch from one to the other is randomized. This design is particularly useful for complex or multifaceted interventions.

A recent example of a high-quality cluster randomized trial was the High-STEACS study[1] which evaluated the use of high-sensitivity cardiac troponin assays to reduce subsequent myocardial infarction or cardiovascular death in patients with suspected acute coronary syndrome. It was a stepped-wedge, cluster-randomized controlled trial across ten secondary or tertiary care hospitals in Scotland. The new assay was compared to conventional troponin testing with five clusters randomized to implementation after an initial validation phase and a 5- to 6-month delay in implementation. The primary outcome was subsequent myocardial infarction or death from cardiovascular causes at 1 year after initial presentation and occurred in 105 (15%) of 720 patients when using standard troponin tests and 131 (12%) of 1051 patients using high-sensitivity assays. This result was not even close to statistical significance ($p = 0.620$) and suggests no important impact of high-sensitivity troponin in these settings.

The choice of trial outcomes is important. It is generally cheaper, due to smaller sample size and reduced follow-up requirements, to use surrogate endpoints. For example, a study of the impact of a cardiovascular risk predictor might use statin prescription or reduction in low-density lipoprotein cholesterol and an endpoint. While the link between each of these and reduced cardiovascular events is well established, a better trial design would follow patients in the trial to determine the number of cardiovascular events in the intervention and control groups.

As discussed earlier, diagnostic strategies do not necessarily need to improve patient outcomes to be worthwhile. Even if outcomes are similar between intervention and control groups, another important benefit can be reduced cost which is studied in cost-effectiveness analysis. A full description of cost-effectiveness analysis is beyond the scope of this book but it should be obvious that within a finite health budget, any intervention that reduces costs without compromising care is likely to be worthwhile.

It is important to keep in mind that the commonest way that tests affect patient outcome is when the information is used to guide decisions to start, withhold, modify, or stop treatment. As a result, the influence of tests is often bound together with the efficacy and side effects of treatments. Put more simply, if tests lead to changes in treatments, the costs and benefits of the treatments need to be considered in trial design. This is expertly explained by Professor Patrick Bossuyt et al. in a *Lancet* paper from 2000.[2] They describe two possible trial designs for determining the impact of Doppler ultrasonography of the umbilical artery in assisting the management of pregnant women with intrauterine growth retardation (IUGR) (Fig. 9.1). While standard of care is to admit all such women to hospital, the hypothesis is that a normal ultrasound scan would allow women to be treated at home. Panel (a) of Fig. 9.1 shows a typical trial design whereby women are randomized to having the ultrasound scan or not having it, and each is followed up to determine the outcome of the pregnancy. At first glance this seems reasonable, if an ultrasound scan is useful in this scenario, pregnancy outcomes of women randomized to ultrasound scans should be better, right? Not necessarily—the issue is that the effectiveness of the intervention, the strategy of managing women at home, has not been tried before and so its efficacy isn't known. What is actually being tested therefore is a test/treatment combination. Look carefully

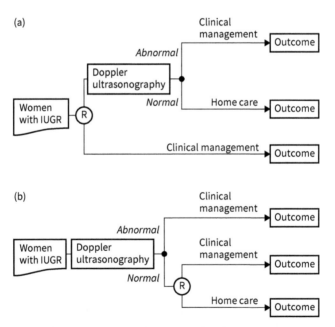

Fig. 9.1 Examples of trial designs to evaluate Doppler ultrasonography (DU) as a new test to improve the care of pregnant women with intrauterine growth retardation (IUGR). (a) Women are randomized (R) to management based on the DU result or standard of care (clinical management). (b) Only women with normal DU are randomized; either to standard of care or management at home. Both trial designs are valid but (b) is much more efficient.

at the diagram and you can see that only women with a normal ultrasound scan con-tribute to the comparison, as all women with an abnormal ultrasound scan, whether in the control or the intervention group, receive the same treatment: admission to hospital. While the study can inform us of the effectiveness of the test/treatment com-bination, it isn't efficient. Panel (b) of Fig. 9.1 shows an alternative design where the point of randomization is shifted to **after** the ultrasound scan. In this case, women with an abnormal ultrasound scan, who didn't contribute to the comparison in the previous design, are excluded and only women with a normal ultrasound scan are randomized. This is a much more efficient design and particularly useful when the test is cheap compared to the follow-up and treatment.

The same paper also discusses the issue of comparing a new diagnostic strategy that might replace the existing standard of care using randomization. The example is the new test of intracoronary flow velocity as a replacement for scintigraphy in deter-mining whether patients with ischaemic heart disease should undergo angiography

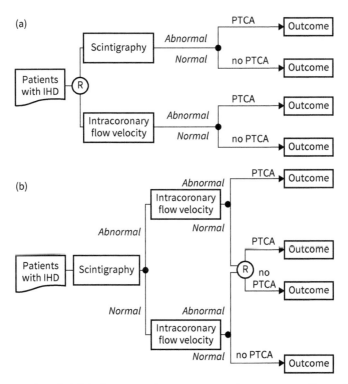

Fig. 9.2 Examples of trial designs to evaluate a new test, intracoronary flow velocity as a replacement for scintigraphy in patients with ischaemic heart disease (IHD). (a) Patients are randomized to one or other of the tests and percutaneous transluminal coronary angiography (PTCA) is performed or not performed depending on the results. (b) All patients have both tests and only those with discordant results are randomized to PTCA or no PTCA. Both trial designs are valid but (b) is much more efficient.

or not. Panel (a) of Fig. 9.2 is the most obvious trial design, that is, randomize parti-cipants to the new or standard of care test, decide whether to perform angiography based on the result, and follow up all patients. This seems sensible but the authors point out that in any participants in whom the two tests agree (both normal or both abnormal), the difference between the groups will be determined by the treatments, not the strategies, and such participants will not contribute to the comparison. A much more efficient design is to apply both strategies to each participant and ran-domize only those with discordant results (e.g. one normal and one abnormal) to the different treatment strategies (panel (b) of Fig. 9.2).

Similar trial designs may not be appropriate or ethical in all circumstances; im-agine a new test for malaria which has been shown in diagnostic accuracy studies to be much more sensitive, and perhaps marginally less specific than the standard of care which is blood smear microscopy. Malaria is often fatal if untreated and so it would not be ethical to randomize a participant with a negative blood smear and a positive novel test to 'no treatment'. Under these circumstances it might be reasonable and effi-cient to randomize only patients with negative blood smears to the new test or no test (clinical judgement). Clearly the design of randomized trials of novel tests is far from obvious and careful consideration of trial design is vital to ensure that studies are eth-ical and efficient.

Notes

1. Shah ASV, Anand A, Strachan FE, Ferry AV, Lee KK, Chapman AR, et al. High-sensitivity troponin in the evaluation of patients with suspected acute coronary syndrome: a stepped-wedge, cluster-randomised controlled trial. Lancet. 2018;392(10151):919–928.
2. Bossuyt PM, Lijmer JG, Mol BW. Randomised comparisons of medical tests: sometimes in-valid, not always efficient. Lancet. 2000;356(9244):1844–1847.

10
Evaluation of a Novel Test

In this chapter, we will draw together everything we have learnt by looking at an example of a diagnostic laboratory test that has recently been introduced and evaluated—a novel test for TB called Xpert MTB/RIF.

TB was designated a global health emergency by the WHO in 1993. In 2019, there were an estimated 10 million cases and 1.4 million deaths worldwide, making it the infectious disease with the greatest mortality burden. In 1882, Robert Koch discovered the aetiology of TB to be infection with *Mycobacterium tuberculosis*, and soon after, Paul Ehrlich developed the first stain for the bacillus and therefore the first diagnostic test. Although staining techniques and microscopes have evolved, the same basic principle of visualizing stained organisms from clinical specimens (usually sputum) is still used today and is called smear microscopy. It remains useful largely because of its low cost and because it is a marker of treatment success, which means that if treatment is working, we see fewer and fewer bacilli on the slide. There are many disadvantages including the need for the patient to produce sputum and for a trained technician. The diagnostic accuracy is highly variable, depending on factors such as operator skill, time spent reading the slide, and patient factors such as age and immune status. During most of the 20th century, typically quoted figures for adults were sensitivity of 80% and specificity of 99%, which equates to likelihood ratios of approximately LR+ve 80 and LR−ve 0.2.

Culture of the organism was developed around the same time as smear microscopy and became the next laboratory test. Again, media and techniques have improved, but the same basic principle is used today—inoculate a culture medium with a patient sample, incubate it, and see if TB grows. In terms of diagnostic accuracy, specificity is considered 100% with LR+ve approaching infinity as a positive culture is usually considered a reference standard. Sensitivity and LR−ve are harder to determine, while a culture will become positive when far fewer bacilli are present, compared to smear microscopy, we know from autopsy studies that patients with multiple negative cultures still die from TB, so sensitivity is not 100% and LR−ve is not 0. Typically, however, when autopsy is not available, multiple negative cultures are considered the reference standard for not having TB in research studies. The main disadvantage of culture, other than cost, is the time it takes for samples to become positive. TB is a slow-growing organism which takes a minimum of around a week but up to 6 weeks to grow in a laboratory, so it takes 6 weeks to be sure that a sample is negative.

Clinical features keeping with TB include persistent cough, drenching night sweats, fever, weight loss, and haemoptysis. CXR is also widely used, with typical features being upper lobe cavities. During most of the 20th century, the combination of history, CXR, smear microscopy, and culture was largely sufficient to diagnose TB. To my knowledge, no formal studies of this strategy were ever conducted and much of this occurred before clinical decision thresholds or likelihood ratios had even been described. However, clinicians were happy with this approach which appeared to be adequate.

Towards of the end of the 20th century, however, things began to change. The driving force was the HIV pandemic. HIV attacks the immune system leaving people increasingly vulnerable to infections and cancers and it turns out that they become particularly susceptible to TB. HIV also changes the clinical presentation of TB in important ways. Firstly, it is more likely to affect organs other than the lungs (extrapulmonary TB), and if it is not in the lungs, sputum is unlikely to be a useful specimen. Secondly, even when the lungs are involved, they are affected in different ways. The weakened immune response is much less likely to produce lung cavities, meaning that CXR findings are less likely to be typical; the patients are less likely to produce sputum and because there are high concentrations of TB bacilli in cavities, smear microscopy is less likely to be positive. Up to 50% of patients with advanced HIV disease and TB are not even able to produce a sputum sample and as a result of the lower bacillary burden, the sensitivity of smear microscopy drops to only around 20%. Thirdly, patients with HIV and untreated TB deteriorate much faster, making the 6-week wait for a culture result too long. Put simply, the patient may have died in that time if you haven't started treatment. In summary, when the HIV pandemic arrived, patients became highly susceptible to TB, they deteriorated much faster, and clinical, radiological, and laboratory diagnostics all performed much worse.

As a result, there was a scramble to develop new laboratory diagnostics that were as accurate as culture but as fast as smear microscopy and preferably could be performed on specimens that were more readily available than sputum. An apparent breakthrough came in 2010 with the publication, in the world's most prestigious medical journal,[1] of a diagnostic accuracy study of a novel assay called Xpert MTB/RIF. The reported sensitivity was 97.6% and specificity of 98.1% when the results of three Xpert MTB/RIF tests on different sputum samples was the index test, and culture of two of these specimens was the reference standard. Importantly, for patients with negative smear microscopy, the sensitivity of a single test was 72.5%, rising to 90.2% when three tests were performed. Laboratory turnaround time is 2 hours, limited technical expertise is required, and there are minimal risks of infecting laboratory workers. Not only that, as an added bonus, the assay can determine resistance to the most important antituberculous drug, rifampicin.[*] On the face of it, this was an impressive result and the WHO endorsed it almost immediately.

---

[*] I would urge you to read and critically appraise this paper. There is a major flaw in the reporting, see if you can spot it. The answer is in Appendix 4.

Multiple studies with similar results followed (we saw the results of a meta-analysis of diagnostic accuracy studies in Chapter 3) and there was a massive roll-out of machines and consumables. Given that TB was (and still is) a global emergency and there had been a clamour for improved diagnostics, this response is understandable. Waiting for diagnostic research (Chapter 8) and diagnostic intervention research (Chapter 9) before implementing the test would have taken too long. However, that research should still have been done.

What actually happened was that the diagnostic research was never adequately performed and investigators essentially skipped that step and jumped directly to diagnostic intervention research. There are now multiple studies with variable designs but sharing the same basic strategy. Randomize participants suspected of TB to diagnosis with Xpert MTB/RIF or smear microscopy then follow them up and measure patient-relevant outcomes such as morbidity and mortality. A systematic review and meta-analyses of these studies published up until 2016 found four suitable studies enrolling a combined total of around 5000 patients.[2] The conclusion is simple: 'Xpert implementation showed no discernible impact on treatment outcomes compared with conventional smear despite reduced time to diagnosis, time to treatment or reduced level of empiric treatment'. A second individual patient data meta-analysis of 8567 outpatients tested for TB in five low-income and middle-income countries was unable to rule in nor rule out a reduction in 6-month all-cause mortality associated with use of Xpert MTB/RIF as an initial diagnostic test, relative to sputum smear microscopy.[3]

This is worth repeating—a new test with much improved diagnostic accuracy, which also determines important drug resistance mutations, when tested in multiple large randomized controlled trials has no effect on morbidity or mortality. Fig. 10.1 is a Forest plot showing no statistically significant effect of Xpert MTB/RIF on favourable outcomes. If this was a new drug rather than a test it would surely be abandoned as ineffective and yet we continue to use Xpert MTB/RIF and its successor Xpert

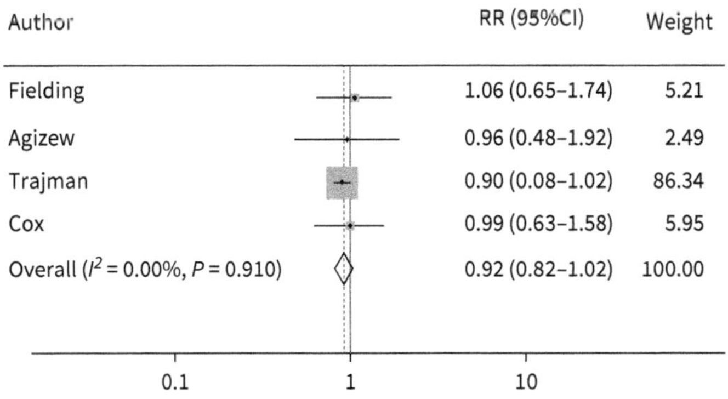

Author		RR (95%CI)	Weight
Fielding		1.06 (0.65–1.74)	5.21
Agizew		0.96 (0.48–1.92)	2.49
Trajman		0.90 (0.08–1.02)	86.34
Cox		0.99 (0.63–1.58)	5.95
Overall (I^2 = 0.00%, P = 0.910)		0.92 (0.82–1.02)	100.00

| | 0.1 | 1 | 10 |

Fig. 10.1 Forest plot showing unfavourable outcomes among tuberculosis patients diagnosed using Xpert MTB/RIF versus smear microscopy. Horizontal axis is relative risk (RR); <1 favours Xpert MTB/RIF, >1 favours smear microscopy.

MTB/RIF Ultra (Ultra) on a wide scale. So, what went wrong, and why are we still using these tests?

In my view, the mistake was to assume that a test with improved diagnostic accuracy would automatically improve outcomes without considering its place within the diagnostic process. In doing so, a great deal of time and money was wasted on inappropriate diagnostic intervention research and we are left not really knowing how to use the test.

An appropriate approach would have been to determine clinical predictors of TB from observational studies and use these to develop prediction rules. Treatment thresholds should have been determined separately. Studies could then have determined which patients had a pre-test probability between test and test–treatment thresholds, and randomized only these patients to Xpert MTB/RIF or smear microscopy.

Clinical prediction rules have subsequently been developed, and we know, for example, that predictors of TB in seriously ill inpatients with HIV include low haemoglobin levels, low or normal white cell count, fever >39°C, >2 weeks' of cough, being unable to walk unaided, and the CXR.[4] Important predictors in outpatients include whether or not the patient is on antiretroviral therapy, number and duration of symptoms, body mass index, and CD4 count. While multiple clinical prediction rules have been proposed, none have been widely validated or are used in routine practice. Nor have clinical decision thresholds been adequately determined in multiple settings.

Intriguingly, a small study recently showed that the best predictor of TB in outpatients with HIV is the judgement of an experienced nurse, which has an unadjusted odds ratio of 6.5. While this is difficult to generalize, it might offer some insight into why randomized studies of Xpert MTB/RIF in outpatients were so disappointing; essentially the nurses (who often are the most senior cadre of staff in low-resource settings) had very good clinical judgement as to which patients had TB. They also knew that negative sputum smear microscopy could not exclude TB in most cases and so correctly initiated many such patients on empiric (without confirmation from a laboratory test) therapy. Had the trials simply asked nurse which patients they were unsure about, and randomized them, the results may well have been different.

Despite the negative trials, the WHO has continued to insist on the widespread roll-out of Xpert MTB/RIF and Ultra. Their 2013 policy update[5] gave a 'strong recommendation based on high-quality evidence' that Xpert MTB/RIF should be used rather than smear microscopy as the initial test in adults suspected of having HIV-associated TB. It is worth delving deeper into why they considered the evidence to be 'high quality' when it appears that in fact the evidence shows a lack of effect. The answer comes by looking at the question they were asking, which was 'What is the diagnostic accuracy of Xpert MTB/RIF for the detection of pulmonary TB in adults, where Xpert MTB/RIF is used as a replacement test for smear microscopy?' As we have seen, there is indeed good evidence of improved diagnostic accuracy, the mistake is to translate improved diagnostic accuracy into improved patient outcomes in the absence of appropriate research. A more appropriate question might have been

'In adults with HIV and suspected TB, does the use of Xpert MTB/RIF when compared to smear microscopy improve patient outcomes?' As we have seen, the answer would be a resounding 'No' based on currently available trials. A better question still might have been 'What is the optimal diagnostic strategy for pulmonary TB in adults with HIV?' Unfortunately, we still don't know the answer to that question. Instead, the WHO has developed target product profiles (TPPs) for new TB tests—these are the expected optimum or minimum diagnostic accuracy that researchers should aim for when developing a new test.[6] The TPP for a test to replace smear microscopy for detecting TB are optimal and minimum sensitivities of >95% and >80%, respectively, and specificity of 98%. For a rapid, biomarker-based, non-sputum-based test to detect TB, overall pooled sensitivity should optimally be ≥80% in adults with HIV infection and minimally ≥65%, whereas specificity should be 98%. You might well ask how the WHO came to these numbers and assume that some complex modelling based on in-depth research was used; in fact, these were merely the consensus of a group of TB scientists who attended a 2-day meeting in Geneva. While the attendees are undoubtedly experts in TB and laboratory testing, it doesn't appear that experts in diagnostic test evaluation were invited.

Having got this far with the book, it should be obvious how unsatisfactory these TPPs are. Firstly, they are defined as sensitivity and specificity alone; secondly, these are merely the consensus agreement of a group of researchers. Unfortunately, there has been very little questioning of these figures and although developed in 2014, researchers continue to try to meet them. It should be clear by now that setting a target for a test based only on diagnostic accuracy is bound to fail. We have already seen, in the TB sphere itself, that improved diagnostic accuracy does not necessarily translate into improved outcomes, and yet the WHO continues to use diagnostic accuracy as a benchmark. It should be clear by now that the utility of a new test is best measured by its impact on patient-relevant outcomes, so a much more appropriate TPP would be something like, in appropriately designed randomized controlled trials, any new test (or diagnostic strategy) should improve morbidity and mortality or decrease cost, when compared to existing tests (or diagnostic strategies).

In summary, there has now been a widespread and costly scale-up of this test despite randomized trials showing no effect on patient-relevant outcomes. However, as a specialist, I routinely use Ultra in my daily practice, either when my clinical judgement is of a pre-test probability between test and test–treatment threshold, or simply to determine the rifampicin resistance status. I remain convinced this test has a place; however, appropriate research has not been done to determine where, when, and how it should be used. As a result, we are struggling to adequately ensure that less experienced clinicians use it appropriately. Despite these failures, the WHO continues to call for tests with improved diagnostic accuracy and sets benchmarks when they should be seeking tests that are shown to improve patient-relevant outcomes and reduce costs.

Notes

1. Boehme C, Nabeta P, Hillemann D, Nicol P, Shenai S, Krapp F, et al. Rapid molecular detection of tuberculosis and rifampin resistance. N Engl J Med. 2010;363(11):1005–1015.
2. Agizew T, Boyd R, Auld AF, Payton L, Pals SL, Lekone P, et al. Treatment outcomes, diagnostic and therapeutic impact: Xpert vs. smear. A systematic review and meta-analysis. Int J Tuberc Lung Dis. 2019;23(1):82–92.
3. Di Tanna GL, Khaki AR, Theron G, McCarthy K, Cox H, Mupfumi L, et al. Effect of Xpert MTB/RIF on clinical outcomes in routine care settings: individual patient data meta-analysis. Lancet Glob Health. 2019;7(2):e191–e199.
4. Griesel R, Stewart A, van der Plas H, Sikhondze W, Rangaka MX, Nicol MP, et al. Clin Infect Dis. 2018;66(9):1419–1426.
5. World Health Organization. Xpert MTB/RIF Assay for the Diagnosis of Pulmonary and Extrapulmonary TB in Adults and Children: Policy Update. Geneva: World Health Organization; 2013. Available at: https://www.who.int/publications/i/item/9789241506335
6. World Health Organization. High-priority Target Product Profiles for New Tuberculosis Diagnostics: Report of a Consensus Meeting. Geneva: World Health Organization; 2014. Available at: https://apps.who.int/iris/bitstream/handle/10665/135617/WHO_HTM_TB_2014.18_eng.pdf

11
Conclusions

The first part of this book discusses the initial evaluation of a novel test and how this might be interpreted when applied to the individual patient we have in front of us. It is written for the medical students and junior doctors who want to be the best they can be. It is likely that expert application of evidence-based medicine to therapies, be they pharmaceutical, surgical, or anything else, will have a bigger impact on morbidity, mortality, and costs. However, testing remains an integral component of all branches of medicine and I would urge you to take pride in your evidence-based approach to this aspect as well. Tests are less rigorously evaluated than therapies, which will make this difficult at times. There won't always be easy ways to calculate pre-test probabilities or find likelihood ratios. There will be even fewer evidence-based examples of thresholds. However, by sticking with the principles outlined in this book you will make fewer mistakes and gradually grow into a competent and confident tester. Below is a suggested four-point plan to consider every time you think of requesting a test.

1. **Formulate a patient-relevant question**. What do you want to know and why do you want to know it? The actions you propose to take after a particular result don't have to be immediate or related to medical or surgical treatments, they can be something you say to a patient or a change in future testing strategy, but they do have to be aimed at improving the physical and/or mental health of the patient or reducing costs.
2. **Calculate whether the test can answer this question**. In diagnostic terms, this means estimating pre-test probability and calculating whether the test can change the probability in a meaningful way, typically by crossing the therapeutic threshold. Similar arguments can be applied to prognostic, monitoring, and other forms of test. For example, the cardiovascular risk of a patient with known age and sex may be known, the question is whether a lipid profile will influence your actions in terms of preventative counselling and/or treatment for preventing cardiovascular disease.
3. **Consider the costs**. Tests typically consume financial and human resources, which might be better used elsewhere. There might be opportunity costs such as delaying effective therapy. Many tests can cause both physical and psychological harm to the patient. Extreme examples are brain biopsies and tests for Huntingdon's disease but taking a blood pressure reading has the potential to

change the prognosis and lifetime treatment plan for a patient. Indirect costs such as misinterpretation of results can be avoided if points 1 and 2 are followed but there can often be uncertainty that must be accounted for.

When calculating the costs, consider the yield. It is fine to perform a test where, for example, a positive result changes management decisions and a negative one doesn't, but when considering the costs, you must bear in mind that a test that is infrequently positive (low yield) is less likely to be cost-effective.

4. **Stop and think**. Weigh up the benefits to the patient (point 2) and the costs (point 3) before making a final decision on the need for the test.

Following this four-point plan won't always be easy. Point 2 in particular may have many uncertainties—pre-test probabilities will often be estimates and likelihood ratios and thresholds may not have been comprehensively studied. However, this should not discourage you from sticking to this framework, which can be applied to almost any scenario. It isn't always easy but you can help yourself by avoiding some **common pitfalls**, listed below:

- 'I just want to know the answer' is rarely (if ever) a valid reason for requesting a test. When clinicians can't develop a patient-relevant question they often resort to saying 'But I just want to know the answer'. The question should then be, but why? There can be valid answers such as 'It will help me with decision-making in future patients if I am sure of the diagnosis in this one', but 'Because I just want to know' is not a valid answer. Medical resources are not available to satisfy these types of cravings by doctors.
- Being a junior doctor can be stressful and tiring. One attempt to make life easier has been the introduction of standardized tick box request forms for investigations, and employment of phlebotomists to draw blood. In many countries, gone are the days when junior doctors wrote out each request form by hand and then took blood themselves. In many ways this is very welcome but it also has the potential to turn rational human beings into tick box zombies, absentmindedly ticking multiple boxes to make sure they 'cover all the bases'. It is possible that junior doctors request more tests than necessary, out of fear of failing to request a test that a senior member of the team may later ask about. This may be compounded by anxiety associated with working in a new team every 4–6 months, after which time junior doctors generally go through the changeover period. My advice is to try to learn from your seniors by asking them if tests you requested were useful to them and which tests they rely heavily on. Don't expect them necessarily to define all their decisions using likelihood ratios and thresholds, but ask them what the patient-relevant questions are in common clinical scenarios and gradually build up your experience and request fewer tests as time goes on.
- Avoid 'double dipping' whenever possible. This refers to requesting multiple tests to answer the same question when a single test already gives you almost all the information you need. For example, alanine transaminase (ALT) is an enzyme

found in the liver that helps convert proteins into energy for the liver cells. When the liver is damaged, ALT is released into the bloodstream and levels increase. Aspartate transaminase (AST) is an enzyme that helps metabolize amino acids; like ALT, its level increases when there is damage to liver cells, but it is also present in many other tissues such as muscle cells and so an increased level may be caused by damage other than to the liver. In other words, AST is less specific to the liver. While there might be some extra information derived from the ratio of the two values, in most instances knowing the AST when you already know the ALT will tell you nothing you didn't already know. A similar argument could be made for measuring urea when you already know the creatinine. It might add information relating to hydration status or gastrointestinal bleeding but very often it won't be helpful.

- Avoid unnecessary repetition of tests. Imagine you measured a full blood count on admission for a patient with fatigue and shortness of breath. You found the haemoglobin concentration to be 5 g/dL, mean corpuscular volume 62 fL, with normal white cell count, differential, and platelets. You transfuse the patient while looking for sites of occult bleeding or other cause of microcytic anaemia. After 2 days you want to measure the haemoglobin again to check the response to the transfusion and to set a new baseline to help determine if there is further bleeding. At this point there is very unlikely to be any abnormality of white cell count or platelets, so why request a full blood count? At this stage a simple haemoglobin will be all that is required.

- Don't put the cart before the horse. 'The procalcitonin is 10, I'm really worried about the patient' is the type of comment I hear commonly from ward doctors. Hopefully it is obvious to you by now what is wrong with this statement. As an infectious diseases doctor, if I want to know the procalcitonin results at all (I rarely do), I want to hear it at the very end of a presentation. First, I want to know the history, examination, vital signs, and other relevant investigations. If the patient is well or improving from an infection point of view, there is very little value in knowing the procalcitonin, so being presented with that value upfront is nonsensical.

  There are of course times when patients are only mildly symptomatic but a test result can be extremely worrying, think of a raised potassium in a patient with renal impairment. In that scenario, 'The potassium is 7.5 and I'm really worried about the patient' is a reasonable comment. However, all too often test results are presented before the clinical condition of the patients which makes no sense.

- Don't use tests that are good for monitoring disease processes (typically with low specificity) to try to make a diagnosis. C-reactive protein (CRP) is a commonly used and relatively well-studied test; for example, it is a useful screening test for TB in asymptomatic adults with HIV and helpful for guiding antibiotic prescription in outpatients with acute exacerbations of COPD. However, it is also commonly requested in patients admitted to hospital with obvious infection, where it is of very little value. Take the common example of an adult with a week of cough and fever, a neutrophilia, and lobar consolidation on their CXR. The diagnosis is CAP and antibiotics are indicated. The value of CRP measurement in this patient is close to zero—yes, there are studies showing that monitoring CRP trends can help decrease antibiotic exposure, but in reality the diagnosis is secure and monitoring can easily be done with daily history taking ('Are you feeling better?'), monitoring fever and respiratory rate. In my own practice of infectious diseases, I have essentially no interest in the CRP of a patient with obvious CAP and if there is another reason that I want to know the result, I'm happy to after-request it and wait for the result.

- Another common example of monitoring tests being requested in order to make a diagnosis is 'tumour markers'. There are a whole range of proteins that can be produced by cancers and measured in the blood or other tissue; these include alpha-feto protein, CA125, and CA19.9. While some may have value in screening highly targeted populations (e.g. alpha-feto protein in patients with chronic hepatitis B at risk of hepatocellular carcinoma), the approach of requesting a 'panel' of tumour markers in patients without a secure diagnosis is likely to fail. It might also create a great deal of distress for a patient if they are told that their tumour marker is high, when in fact it is of very little significance.

The second half of this book describes the evaluation of tests from a public health perspective and poses the question 'What evidence is required for a test to be recommended for use within a health system?' As with the evaluation of tests on individuals, much of the important research remains to be done. However, it is important to understand that, as with drugs, tests have side effects and costs, which mean that a thorough evidence-based approach is required before they can be recommended for use.

News headlines are generally a poor guide to medical advances but it can be interesting to look at these and think through the evaluations you would like to perform. An almost random example is a headline in my news feed this morning which reads 'Pitchside saliva test to diagnose concussion has "game-changing" trial'. If I have written the book I hope to have written, a number of questions will immediately spring to mind and you will be keen to read the scientific manuscript from the study. The story goes on to describe a test using microscopic DNA markers with an accuracy of 94%, which is variously described as a 'breakthrough' and 'incredibly exciting'. You will want to know the domain that was studied (elite male rugby union players) and the reference standard for concussion. This is the Head Injury Assessment (HIA), which is performed by a doctor when a player with a potential head injury is temporarily removed from the pitch. The doctor typically uses the current version of the Sports Concussion Assessment Tool (SCAT), which involves physical examination and tests of cognitive function such as asking the venue of the game and which team scored last. You would then like to know more about the index test and how it was performed. Then you would like to see the 2×2 table to find out where those 6% of false tests lie. In this context, false-negative index tests (low sensitivity and NPV and high LR–ve) are likely to be much more worrying than false positives because the implications of a concussed rugby player returning to the field are greater than a non-concussed player being removed from the game. You would like to see that the study is published according to the STARD guideline and check each feature for yourself. Even if the study is large, of high quality, and shows no false negatives, you will be hesitant to conclude that it is a 'game changer'. You would be interested in the costs of a HIA and how these might be reduced by the index test. The HIA is currently cheap, if the presence of a doctor is required at pitch side for other purposes, so the introduction of the novel test might increase costs. Perhaps there are other advantages such as speed; the current HIA takes 10 minutes, and perhaps the index test reduces this appreciably. You would also like to see more research in other domains, such as elite female rugby union players or similar high-velocity impact sports. All in all, you will be highly sceptical of this headline when you first read it, knowing that newspapers and even scientific reporters are prone to hyperbole and that a thorough evaluation of the study is necessary.

In 2020, the BBC was one of many news outlets to run stories on dogs that are trained to sniff out COVID-19. In one particular video, the researcher claimed 'almost 100% accuracy'. The video goes on to show dogs moving between cones which each have an item of clothing at the smaller end. The dog sniffs each one in turn and sits down next to the cone with clothing from the COVID-19 patient. As a news story this seems quite impressive. Imagine a dog walking around and airport picking out people with COVID-19 before they board their plane; or perhaps walking down a line of people at a clinic and making the diagnosis without the need for a swab and a laboratory test.

This is another example of a newsworthy story making headlines long before appropriate studies have been done. It will be fairly obvious to you at this point what the limitations of this approach are. To begin with, placing single items of clothing in cone devices in a laboratory is completely unlike the real-world settings in which the test might be useful. In reality, an airport is full of thousands of smells, sights, and sounds that might distract the dog.

So, while it's absolutely fine for researchers to begin with this type of study to try to pick up a signal, nobody should get carried away when they see that dogs can make this judgement in such a controlled environment.

To conclude, we will return to where we began and examine the thought process of the shrewd professor and a naïve medical registrar. As a reminder, we were reviewing an 18-year-old woman with 6 months of secondary amenorrhea, a negative urinary pregnancy test, and mildly raised prolactin. Both the GP and the medical registrar (me) thought that prolactinoma was likely. The professor asked for a repeat pregnancy test, and that was positive. While I was in a conundrum, the professor diagnosed pregnancy and moved to the next patient. So how exactly did she get to the correct answer so efficiently and why was I still confused?

My approximate thought process is captured in the three Fagan nomograms in Fig. 11.1. Note that the post-test probability after one test becomes the pre-test probability

88

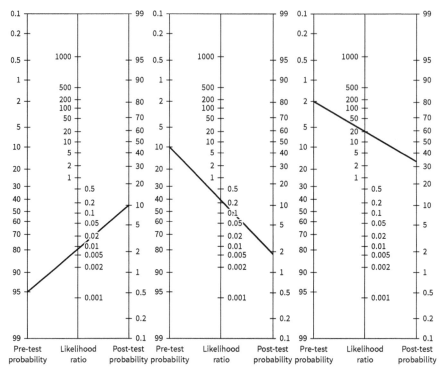

Fig. 11.1 Three Fagan nomograms illustrating the author's thinking with regard to pregnancy in an amenorrhoeic, sexually active 18-year-old female. Left panel, pre-test probability 95% with negative pregnancy test gives post-test probability 10%. Middle panel, probability drops to 2% based on mildly raised prolactin. Right panel, probability increases to 35% based on positive pregnancy test.

for the next. To begin with, I assumed that an amenorrhoeic 18-year-old female who was sexually active with a man, not using any form of contraception, and had no other obvious causes for amenorrhea had a pre-test probability of pregnancy of around 95%. I then interpreted the first pregnancy test by assuming a LR−ve of around 0.01 and arrived at a post-test probability of 10% (left hand nomogram). I then assumed that because the raised prolactin was consistent with prolactinoma, then the likelihood ratio with respect to pregnancy was negative. Using LR−ve = 0.2 I arrived at a post-test probability of 2%. For the second pregnancy test I then used LR+ve = 20 and arrived at a final probability of pregnancy of 33%. This value was between the test (1%) and test-treatment (99%) thresholds I had set and so I wanted to perform more tests.

Of course, in the moment I wasn't actually thinking in likelihood ratios, probabilities, and thresholds. In reality I was putting together all the information in my head: the history, examination, and three tests performed in series to get to the point where I was unsure of the diagnosis. This can be illustrated with a single Fagan nomogram (Fig. 11.2) as the three likelihood ratios I ascribed can be multiplied to give

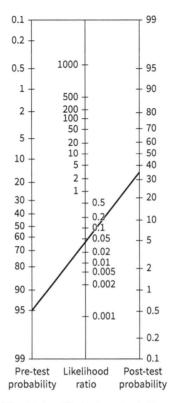

Fig. 11.2 The three tests of Fig. 11.1 unified into a single Fagan nomogram.

a single value (0.01×0.2×20 = 0.04). Using the pre-test probability of 95% and this single likelihood ratio also gives a post-test probability of 33%.

Let's now turn to the professor and her thinking, which is illustrated in the three Fagan nomograms in Fig. 11.3. She also began with 95% pre-test probability but correctly interpreted the first pregnancy test, using LR–ve = 0.08 to give a post-test probability of 50%. She then knew that the mildly raised prolactin was in favour of pregnancy and therefore the likelihood ratio was >1. She calculated the probability of pregnancy after the prolactin result to be 85% using LR+ve = 5. The second pregnancy test was then simple to interpret, leading to >99% probability (LR+ve = 20). This was easily above the test–treatment threshold and so she was happy to make the diagnosis without further tests.

So, was the professor formally calculating probabilities and likelihood ratios to get to the answer? I doubt it very much. More likely she was using her superior experience and knowledge to combine all the information and arrive at the correct result. This can also be illustrated with a single Fagan nomogram with a combined likelihood ratio of 8 (Fig. 11.4).

The point is that it might well have taken her 20 years to get to this point; she might have encountered several similar situations before, with each one adding to

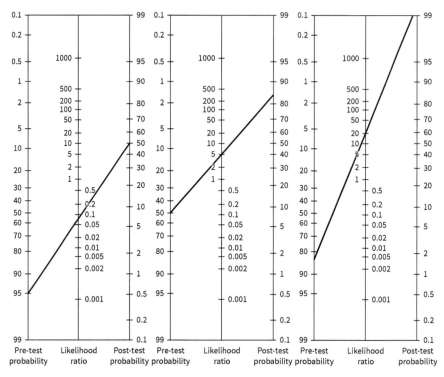

Fig. 11.3 Three Fagan nomograms illustrating the shrewd professor's thinking with regard to pregnancy in an amenorrhoeic, sexually active 18-year-old female. Left panel, pre-test probability 95% with negative pregnancy test gives post-test probability 50%. Middle panel, probability **increases** 85% based on mildly raised prolactin. Right panel, probability increases to >99% based on positive pregnancy test.

her experience until she got to this point. The reason for learning about Bayesian thinking as an inexperienced doctor is that it is a window into the mind of the more experienced. You are not obliged to formally calculate probabilities using calculators on your phone, although this will help. Instead, when an experienced clinician befuddles you with their decision-making, go back and analyse the situation, as I have done above. Try to work out what their thinking was—it probably won't help to ask them what likelihood ratios they were using but ask them how much each piece of information influenced their thinking and in which direction. This will aid your learning and help you reach the level of the professor faster than you ever thought possible.

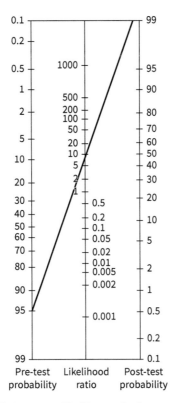

Fig. 11.4 The three tests of Fig. 11.3 unified into a single Fagan nomogram.

The Reverend Thomas Bayes and the Monty Hall Problem

Thomas Bayes (1701–7 April 1761) was an English statistician, philosopher, and Presbyterian minister whose most famous work 'Bayes' theorem' was only published after his death. His solution to a problem of inverse probability was presented in 'An Essay towards solving a Problem in the Doctrine of Chances' which was read to the Royal Society in 1763, 2 years after his death. Richard Price shepherded the work through this presentation and its publication in the *Philosophical Transactions of the Royal Society of London* the following year. Bayes' theorem describes the probability of an event, based on prior knowledge of conditions that might be related to the event.

The Monty Hall problem is a brain teaser based on the concept of Bayes' theorem, in the form of a probability puzzle, loosely based on the American television game show *Let's Make a Deal* and named after its original host, Monty Hall.

In a 1990 letter by Craig Whitaker to Marilyn vos Savant's 'Ask Marilyn' column in *Parade* he asked:

> Suppose you're on a game show, and you're given the choice of three doors: behind one door is a car; behind the others, goats. You pick a door, say No. 1, and the host, who knows what's behind the doors, opens another door, say No. 3, which has a goat. He then says to you, 'Do you want to pick door No. 2?' Is it to your advantage to switch your choice?

Vos Savant's response was that the contestant should switch to the other door. Under the standard assumptions, contestants who switch have a 2/3 chance of winning the car, while contestants who stick to their initial choice have only a 1/3 chance.

Many readers of vos Savant's column refused to believe switching is beneficial despite her explanation. After the problem appeared in *Parade*, approximately 10,000 readers, including nearly 1000 with PhDs, wrote to the magazine, most of them claiming vos Savant was wrong. Even when given explanations, simulations, and formal mathematical proofs, many people still did not accept that switching is the best strategy. Paul Erdős, one of the most prolific mathematicians in history, remained unconvinced until he was shown a computer simulation demonstrating vos Savant's predicted result.

If you remain unconvinced, perhaps try a simulation yourself by having a friend play the role of the quizmaster. She places a coin under one of three unturned cups. You choose a cup and she removes one of the two remaining cups that does not have the coin. You won't be surprised that if you keep your cup and repeat many times, on 1/3 of occasions you will have chosen the coin. Now repeat the process many times but switch to the remaining cup each time and count how often you end up with the coin. You will quickly realize that you end up with the coin twice as often, 2/3 of the time.

This is a practical demonstration of Bayes' theorem. Your prior odds (akin to pre-test probability) of choosing a cup with a coin is 1/3. By removing a cup without a coin, the quiz master is adding information, essentially multiplying that probability by a Bayes factor (akin to a likelihood ratio). The probability that the remaining cup has a coin increases to 2/3, and it now makes sense to switch.

APPENDIX 2

Updating Probabilities Using Bayes' Theorem

This is a worked example where pre-test probability is 10% and LR+ve 24.75.
The first step is to convert the probability to odds:

$$\text{Odds} = \text{probability} / (1 - \text{probability})$$
$$\text{Probability} = 0.1 \ (10\%)$$
$$\text{So odds} = 0.1/(1 - 0.1) = 0.111111$$

The next step is to multiply the odds by LR+ve:

$$0.111111 \times 24.75 = 2.76$$

Then we must convert odds back to probability:

$$\text{Probability} = \text{odds} / (1 + \text{odds})$$
$$\text{So post} - \text{test probability} = 2.76 / (1 + 2.76) = 0.735 \ (74\%)$$

APPENDIX 3

Therapeutic Threshold

The equation for the therapeutic threshold (Tth) is:

$$Tth = C / C + B$$

where:

B = treating disease (survival after a laparotomy for appendicitis) – not treating disease (survival after appendicitis not treated with laparotomy) = 99.9% – 99% = 0.9%

C = not treating no disease (not performing a laparotomy when there is no appendicitis) – treating no disease (performing a laparotomy when there is no appendicitis) = 100% – 99.9% = 0.1%

Therefore:

$$Tth = 0.1/0.9 + 0.1 = 0.1 = 10\%$$

Critical Appraisal of
Boehme et al N Engl J Med 2010

If you examine the paper carefully you will see that diagnostic accuracy is reported as sensitivity of 97.6% and specificity of 98.1%, which equates to LR+ve 51 and LR−ve 0.02. This is based on any of three sputum samples, two were tested with liquid culture and all three tested with Xpert MTB/RIF. The reference standard for TB was any culture positive and for the index test any Xpert MTB/RIF positive. Look carefully and you will also see that the 105 patients with 'clinical tuberculosis' who were culture negative were excluded from this analysis; 31 were index test positive and 74 negative.

There is no scientific justification for excluding these patients. While the STARD criteria had not been published at this time, it would clearly be termed an 'inappropriate exclusion' and the editors of the world's top medical journal should have picked it up. The 105 participants were all culture negative from two samples so would fulfil the reference standard for not having TB. A simple recalculation including this group, gives a specificity of 94% and LR+ve 16. Using a realistic pre-test probability for outpatients of 5%, this equates to a reduction in post-test probability from 73% to only 46%. This is an important change, and could be the difference between initiating and not initiating therapy for many patients with a potentially large public health impact.

Similar mistakes have not been repeated in all diagnostic accuracy studies of Xpert MTB/ RIF. However, this is a reminder that even when published in the most reputable of journals, it is vital to read papers thoroughly as mistakes can still be apparent.

Further Reading

Many of the important resources are included as references within the book. Rather than list further articles, I would rather direct you to people who are giants of the field. If you are interested in further reading try searching for their names; I can pretty much guarantee that if any of the following people have attached their names to an article or book chapter it will be worth reading. This list is not exhaustive by any means so you could also take a so-called snowball approach by searching for work by their co-authors, who might not appear on my list, but are likely to have produced high-quality work.

In no particular order:

Karel G. M. Moons, Julius Center for Health Sciences and Primary Care, University Medical Center Utrecht, Str. 6.131, PO Box 85500, 3508 GA Utrecht, The Netherlands.

Douglas G. Altman (deceased).

Johannes B. Reitsma, Julius Center for Health Sciences and Primary Care, University Medical Center Utrecht, Str. 6.131, PO Box 85500, 3508 GA Utrecht, The Netherlands.

Gary S. Collins, Centre for Statistics in Medicine, Nuffield Department of Orthopaedics, Rheumatology and Musculoskeletal Sciences, University of Oxford, Oxford, UK.

Richard D. Riley, Research Institute for Primary Care and Health Sciences, Keele University, Staffordshire, UK.

Patrick M. Bossuyt, Department of Clinical Epidemiology and Biostatistics, Academic Medical Center, University of Amsterdam, 1100 DE Amsterdam, The Netherlands.

Paul Glasziou, Centre for Evidence-Based Medicine, Department of Primary Health Care, University of Oxford, Oxford, UK.

Jonathan J. Deeks, Public Health, Epidemiology and Biostatistics, University of Birmingham, Edgbaston, Birmingham, UK.

Andre-Pascal Kengne, South African Medical Research Council, Francie Van Zijl Drive, Parow Valley, Cape Town, 7501, South Africa.

Index

For the benefit of digital users, indexed terms that span two pages (e.g., 52–53) may, on occasion, appear on only one of those pages.